Springer

Tokyo
Berlin
Heidelberg
New York
Hong Kong
London
Milan
Paris

M. Onji

Dendritic Cells
in Clinics

With 28 Figures, Including 9 in Color

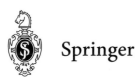 Springer

Morikazu Onji, M.D., Ph.D.
Chairperson and Professor
Third Department of Internal Medicine
Ehime University School of Medicine
454 Shitsukawa, Shigenobu-cho, Onsen-gun, Ehime 791-0295, Japan

ISBN 4-431-40198-9 Springer-Verlag Tokyo Berlin Heidelberg New York

Library of Congress Cataloging-in-Publication Data

Onji, M. (Morikazu), 1948–
    Dendritic cells in clinics / M. Onji.
        p.   ;   cm.
    Includes bibliographical references and index.
    ISBN 4-431-40198-9 (alk. paper)
    1. Dendritic cells.   I. Title.
    [DNLM: 1. Dendritic Cells–immunology.   2. Dendritic Cells–physiology. QW 568 O58d 2004]
    QR185.8.D45O54 2004
    616.07′9—dc22

                                                                2003065717

Printed on acid-free paper

Springer-Verlag is a part of Springer Science+Business Media
springeronline.com

Typesetting: SNP Best-set Typesetter Ltd., Hong Kong
Printing and binding: Nikkei Printing Inc., Japan
SPIN: 10932490

I dedicate this book to my mentor,
the late Professor Yasuyuki Ohta.
The publication of this work was possible only with
the encouragement and support of my wife, Yoshie.

Foreword

The past decade has seen an exponential growth in basic and applied dendritic cell biology. This rapid expansion in knowledge reflects the extraordinary importance attached to these rare, uniquely well-equipped, antigen-presenting leukocytes as inducers and regulators of immune reactivity. Their ability to act as sentinels and as nature's immunologic adjuvants on the one hand, and as instruments of self-tolerance on the other, reflects a remarkable functional plasticity. A great deal of insight has recently been gained into the functional dichotomy of dendritic cells that appears to reflect their stage of maturation and their hematopoietic lineage affiliation. Furthermore, an increasing number of dendritic cell subsets has been identified in both mice and humans. Thus, in addition to the classic myeloid dendritic cells identified by Steinman and Cohn in 1973, both Langerhans cells (the specialized dendritic cells of the epidermis) and so-called plasmacytoid dendritic cells have now been well characterized. Much of the excitement that this evolving and complex picture of dendritic cell biology has generated is linked to the potential of these cells for treating cancer and infectious disease and, conversely, for the treatment of adverse immune reactions (autoimmune disorders, transplant rejection, and allergy). It is fitting that Professor Onji and his colleagues, Drs. Akbar and Horiike, have written this informative and timely text for clinicians and basic immunologists. They have been pioneers and leaders in the study of dendritic cells in relation to liver disease and its therapy. The book will be especially valuable to those who wish to apprise themselves of the important translational aspects of dendritic cell biology, as discoveries in the laboratory are applied in the clinic. It is my pleasure to be associated with this book and to write this foreword.

Angus W. Thomson, Ph.D., D.Sc.
Professor of Surgery and Immunology
University of Pittsburgh Medical Center
Pittsburgh, PA, U.S.A.
October 1, 2003

Preface

The year Steinman and Cohn discovered the "modern-day" dendritic cell in 1973, I graduated from medical school. The Ehime University School of Medicine that has provided me with an excellent academic atmosphere for the last 26 years was established that same year. Significantly for me, 2003 is the 10th anniversary of my becoming professor and chairperson of the school's Third Department of Internal Medicine. The publication of *Dendritic Cells in Clinics* is a personal landmark, reminding me that a lot of valuable time has passed. To that end, the Alumni Association of the Third Department of Internal Medicine (known affectionately as the Yellow Orchid Club in English and as *Ourankai* in Japanese) has provided all sorts of support for its publication.

The principal aim of this book is to provide comprehensive and up-to-date information about dendritic-cell research to clinicians and young clinical immunologists, who encounter these cells either in the laboratory or in patients. Rapid progress has been made over the last 10 years, and dendritic cells are no longer seen as jockeying for position as antigen-presenters; rather, they have received universal recognition as the initiators and regulators of the immune system. They recognize the abnormal, the non-self, and the dangerous and present small amounts of antigen to the lymphocytes. Dendritic cells also induce immunogenic tolerance and are at the forefront of the maintenance of homeostasis by controlling autoimmunity and allergic reactions. They also play a role in transplantation, with a subset of dendritic cells producing high amounts of type-1 interferon, as well as influencing the functions of natural killer cells and macrophages.

My first encounter with the term "dendritic cells" came from a chance observation in 1988, when one of my colleagues, a young doctor, detected hepatitis B surface antigen on follicular dendritic cells in the lymphoid follicles in the portal areas of patients with chronic hepatitis B. Subsequently, I came to discover antigen-presenting dendritic cells and became excited about the enormous potential of dendritic cells in clinical immunology, particularly in the context of autoimmune liver diseases and viral hepatitis. The study of these diseases is both my main research interest and my life's work.

Dr. Sk. Md. Fazle Akbar, who demonstrated the impaired function of dendritic cells in hepatitis B virus carriers for his Ph.D. thesis in the early 1990s, was the first of my colleagues to analyze antigen-presenting dendritic cells. Since then, more than 10 of us have studied different aspects of dendritic cells in liver and gastrointestinal diseases. The manuscripts arising from our departmental research about dendritic cells can be found at the end of the book.

It is now possible to get many kinds of dendritic cell from human peripheral blood, and clinicians are no longer working on the feasibility of dendritic cell-based therapy, but are busy working toward the qualitative improvement of the therapy in malignancies, chronic infection, allergic diseases, autoimmune diseases, and transplantation.

I have a tremendous affection for dendritic cells, mainly due to their shape, phenotypic plasticity, and functional diversity. Their nature resembles the progress of human civilization in many ways. One of the most important aspects of society is how we interact with others. Dendritic cells also move around, meeting, encountering, and interacting with antigens and cells—self and non-self, dangerous and harmful. The information that dendritic cells receive from these encounters is transmitted to other immune-system cells. The outcome of these interactions is the growth, activation, and maturation of dendritic cells and their partners. I am confident that this book will give readers an opportunity to interact with dendritic cells, which will ultimately lead to their individual growth and the benefit of humanity in general.

I would like to acknowledge my gratefulness to the President of the Yellow Orchid Club, Dr. Naofumi Oono, and the 258 active members of the club for their cooperation in writing this book and also for their sustained cooperation as I continue investigating dendritic cells.

Ever forward, steady in the wind.

Morikazu Onji, September 2003

Contents

Includes sources for figure citations

List of Abbreviations

Ab	Antibody
ACBP	Acyl-CoA-binding protein
AD	Atopic dermatitis
Ag	Antigen
AIH	Autoimmune hepatitis
Anti-BDCA	Antibody to blood dendritic cell antigen
Anti-HBs	Antibody to HBsAg
APC	Antigen-presenting cell
BAFF	B-cell activating factor belonging to the TNF family
BCR	B-cell receptor complex
BDCA	Blood dendritic cell antigen
CCR	CC chemokine receptor
CD	Cluster of differentiation
CFA	Complete Freund's adjuvant
CH-B	Chronic hepatitis B
CH-C	Chronic hepatitis C
CLA	Cutaneous leukocyte antigen
CLP	Common lymphoid progenitor
CMP	Common myeloid progenitor
CMV	Cytomegalovirus
Con A	Concanavalin A
CTL	Cytotoxic T lymphocyte
CTLA	Cytotoxic T lymphocyte-associated antigen
CXCR	CX chemokine receptor
DC	Dendritic cell
DC-LAMP	Dendritic cell lysosome-associated membrane protein
DC-SIGN	DC-specific ICAM-3-grabbing nonintegrin
DDC	Dermal dendritic cell
DM	Diabetes mellitus
DNA	Deoxyribonuclic acid
EBV	Epstein-Barr virus
FABP	Fatty acid-binding protein
FDC	Follicular dendritic cell
Flt-3L	fms-like tyrosine kinase receptor 3 ligand
FXVIIIa	Intracytoplasmic trnsglutaminase clotting factor VIIIa

GCDC	Germinal center DC
G-CSF	Granulocyte colony stimulating factor
GM-CSF	Granulocyte-macrophage colony-stimulating factor
gp	Glycoprotein
HBeAg	Hepatitis B e antigen
HBsAg	Hepatitis B surface antigen
HBV	Hepatitis B virus
HCC	Hepatocellular carcinoma
HCV	Hepatitis C virus
HEV	High endothelial venule
HIV	Human immunodeficiency virus
HPC	Hematopoietic progenitor cell
HSC	Hematopoietic stem cell
hsp	Heat shock protein
ICAM	Intracellular adhesion molecule
Id	Inhibitor of DNA binding
IDC	Interdigitating dendritic cell
IFN	Interferon
Ig	Immunoglobulin
IL	Interleukin
ILT	Immunoglobulin-like transcript
IRF	Interferon regulatory factor
KLH	Keyhole limpet hemocyanin
L	Ligand
LAM	Lipoarabinomannan
LAMP	Lysosome-associated membrane protein
LC	Langerhans cell
LCMV	Lymphocytic choriomeningitis virus
LFA	Lymphocyte function-associated protein
LP	Lamina propria
LPS	Lipopolysaccharide
LT	Lymphotoxin
MIIC	MHC class II-rich compartment
mAb	Monoclonal antibody
M-CSF	Macrophage colony stimulating factor
MHC	Major histocompatibility complex
MICA/B	MHC class I-related chains A and B
MIF	Macrophage migration inhibitory factor
MIP	Macrophage inflammatory protein
MV	Measles virus
MLR	Mixed leukocyte/lymphocyte reaction
MRP	Myeloid-related protein
MyD88	Myeloid differentiation marker 88
NF-κB	Nuclear factor kappa B
NIPC	Natural interferon-producing cell
NK	Natural killer
NKT	Natural killer T cell

NLDC	Nonlymphoid dendritic cell
NO	Nitric oxide
NOD	Nonobese diabetic
NPC	Nonparenchymal cell
ODN	Oligodeoxynucleotide
PALS	Periarteriolar lymphatic sheath
PBC	Primary biliary cirrhosis
PBDC	Peripheral blood DC
PBL	Peripheral blood lymphocyte
PBMC	Peripheral blood mononuclear cell
PCR	Polymerase chain reaction
PDC	Pyruvate dehydrogenase complex
PP	Peyer's patch
PrPres	Protease-resistant prion
PSA	Prostate-specific antigen
R	Receptor
RANK	Receptor activator of nuclear factor kappa B
RBC	Red blood corpuscle
RNA	Ribonucleic acid
SACS	*Staphylococcus aureus* Cowan strain
SCF	Stem cell factor
SIV	Simian immunodeficiency virus
SLA	Swine leukocyte antigen
SLC	Secondary lymphoid-tissue chemokine
SLE	Systemic lupus erythematosus
TAA	Tumor-associated antigen
TAP	Transporter-associated antigen processing
TCR	T-cell receptor
Tg	Transgenic
TGF	Transforming growth factor
Th	T helper
TLR	Toll-like receptor
TNF	Tumor necrosis factor
TNFR	Tumor necrosis factor receptor
T^{Reg}	T Regulatory
UC	Ulcerative colitis
VCAM	Vascular cell adhesion molecule
VSV	Vascular stomatitis virus

1. History and Concept of Dendritic Cells

Discovery to Clinical Applications

In 1868, medical student Paul Langerhans discovered a population of dendritically shaped cells in the suprabasal region of the epidermis. These cells now bear his name. The reactivity of these cells to gold salt made him believe that they represented sensory nerve endings. However, today we know that Langerhans cells (LCs) are dendritic leukocytes, which perform a variety of activities; in particular, they function as professional antigen-presenting cells (APCs).

During the 1960s, a consensus developed among immunologists that three cell types, T lymphocytes, B lymphocytes, and macrophages, collaborate during the induction of an antigen (Ag)-specific immune response. The role of B lymphocytes in the production of antibodies was already known, and it was also clear that T lymphocytes played a dominant role in the induction of cell-mediated immunity. Nevertheless, there were several black holes regarding the mechanism of T cell-mediated cellular immune responses. Two factors were mainly responsible for this state of affairs. First, it was known that T lymphocytes are devoid of receptors for microbial agents or tumor cells, so it was unclear how T lymphocytes could interact with these agents without having such receptors. Second, T lymphocytes are not equipped with apparatuses for capturing and internalizing microbes or their Ags, which is essential for the induction of Ag-specific immunity. Thus, it was speculated that, in addition to T lymphocytes, there should be one or more additional types of specialized cells in the immune system that would be capable of capturing, internalizing, and processing microbes or their Ags in situ. Traditionally, cells with these characteristics are referred to as APCs.

The responsibility for the uptake of microbes or their Ags was on the shoulders of macrophages, and these were the primary cells recognized as APCs until 1973, when Ralph Steinman and Zanvil Cohn proposed that a new type of cell, the dendritic cell (DC), functioned as an APC in immunology. They isolated and characterized these novel immunocytes from mouse spleen. DCs were larger than classical lymphocytes, had rough surfaces, and lacked some of the characteristic features of macrophages. Phase contrast microscopy revealed many dendritic processes on their surfaces. Spleen DCs were not shown at this time to express surface markers for lymphocyte or monocyte lineages, but the technical limitations of the early 1970s should be borne in mind. Spleen DCs were motile and expressed very high levels of major histocompatibility complex (MHC) class I and II antigens. Functional analyses revealed that

1

spleen DCs were highly potent stimulators of autologous and allogenic T lymphocytes in vitro. DCs adhered to the plastic surface initially, but became nonadherent after overnight culture. This unique property of spleen DCs, along with their shape, motility, absence of phagocytic apparatuses, and potent allostimulatory capacity, gave Steinman the scientific and logical basis to consider these cells to constitute a novel cell population.

In time, new surface markers for DCs were identified and new functions of DCs revealed. Potent Ag-capturing apparatuses of DCs were also evident. Gradually, DCs gained recognition as APCs. DCs were localized, enriched, and isolated from other lymphoid and nonlymphoid tissues, including blood, lymph, thymus, and bone marrow. The functions of DCs in these tissues and organs were also characterized. During the 10 years or so from the discovery of spleen DCs in 1973 until the mid-1980s, DC studies were dominated by immunologists. Few clinicians were interested in DCs, because the concept of APCs was not clear in physiological or pathological contexts. It was even unknown whether APCs played any role in the pathogenesis of immune-mediated diseases, persistent infections, or malignancies. Although lymphocytes occupied a central position in different immunological events, little experimental evidence was available regarding the direct roles of lymphocytes in pathological conditions. The development of immune therapies for pathological conditions was limited to activating lymphocytes in vivo by immune modulatory agents or the administration of lymphocytes activated in vitro. Needless to say, DC-based therapy was not even dreamed of by clinicians.

Beginning in the mid-1980s, some important developments in this field drew the attention of clinicians to APCs and DCs. Using immunohistochemical methods, some investigators detected DCs or DC-like cells at the site of pathological lesions in some human diseases. Furthermore, the prognosis of some diseases was related to the frequency of infiltrated DCs in the pathological tissues: the more DCs were present in the tissues, the better the prognosis was. By this time, a consensus had developed among immunologists regarding the roles of APCs during the induction of Ag-specific immune responses. The roles of DCs in the pathogenesis of diseases and the potential scope of DC-based therapies for treating pathological conditions started to become evident about this time.

It became evident that many pathological conditions might relate to the defective functioning of APCs or DCs. Researchers started to find some answers to questions that had long been unanswerable by the conventional wisdom. Clinicians started to ask why some patients suffering from chronic microbial infections were unable to mount an effective immune response against the microbes in vivo, even though there were abundant amounts of microbial agents and their Ags in the sera and tissues of these patients, nor was an immune response to microbe-encoded Ags seen in vitro. Interestingly, these patients did not show any features of a generalized immune deficiency, indicating that a very specific defect in the handling of microbial agents or their Ags might be present in these patients. Historically, this problem had been attributed to defective induction, production, or functioning of microbe- or microbial Ag-specific lymphocytes. However, DC researchers showed that the production of Ag-specific lymphocytes was dependent mostly on the recognition, processing, and presentation of Ags to lymphocytes by DCs. Clinicians started to predict that defective APC functioning of DCs might account for the impaired formation of Ag-specific lymphocytes in patients with persistent microbial infections. The next step was comparatively easier; improvement of the functioning of DCs in vivo in these patients might have therapeutic benefits.

Whereas impaired functioning of DCs was a matter of concern for clinicians dealing with persistent microbial infections, the opposite was true for transplant specialists. The induction of an immune response to alloantigens is related to the rejection of transplanted organs. As DCs are the most potent stimulator of allogenic lymphocytes, a role for DCs in the context of transplant acceptance or rejection was predicted. It was postulated that if the immune modulatory capacity of DCs could be down-regulated or if tolerogenic DCs could be propagated in vivo, the chances of acceptance of transplanted organs might be increased.

Clinicians dealing with allergy and autoimmunity also found that DCs might play important roles in these conditions. At this time, the role of DCs as regulators of the immune response became evident. DCs were capable of polarizing T lymphocytes toward either T helper (Th) 1 or Th2 types of immune responses, depending on the nature of the Ag, the antigen dose, the duration of the ligation with T cells, and the availability of cytokines in the tissue microenvironment. Clinicians dealing with allergic diseases suspected that DCs might play a role in Th2 polarization in the context of immunity against allergens. The scope of therapies targeting DCs for allergic conditions was expanded.

One of the main functions of DCs under physiological conditions is to induce immunogenic tolerance to self-antigens and harmless entities. Moreover, DCs play potent roles in inducing and controlling central and peripheral tolerance. Impaired functioning of DCs in genetically susceptible hosts might induce and perpetuate autoimmunity. Many clinicians became interested in regulating the functioning of DCs in vivo to handle autoimmune diseases.

For a long time, it was known that tumors somehow avoid the normal immune surveillance system, leading to uncontrolled growth of tumors. It remained unknown, however, why tumors were able to escape from this surveillance. DCs should bear the primary responsibility for recognizing tumors, and they would also be expected to induce innate and adaptive immunity against tumors. The uncontrolled growth of tumors, therefore, indicates some impairment in the functioning of DCs in tumor-bearing patients. Several investigators had been able to show impaired functioning of DCs in almost all types of human and animal tumors. New information was accumulating regarding the nature of the defect in the DCs of tumor-bearing hosts. During 1990s, several tumor-associated antigens (TAAs) were also discovered. This led to the use of TAA-pulsed DCs for the treatment of tumors.

The most important clinical breakthrough regarding DCs was the development of techniques to enrich DCs from human peripheral blood. Various studies had reported the enrichment of DCs from human blood by several methodologies, but the real breakthrough in this area came when abundant DCs were produced by culturing an adherent population of human peripheral blood mononuclear cells with a cocktail of cytokines. This initiated a series of functional studies using blood DCs from patients with different pathological conditions.

From 1973 to the late 1990s, the roles of DCs were evaluated mainly in the context of the induction of adaptive immune responses. In 1999, some reports showed that DCs are not only related to adaptive immunity; a subset of DC precursors are potent producers of type-1 interferon (IFN). These DC precursors are called natural IFN-producing cells (NIPCs). In addition to their potent capacity to produce type-1 IFN, they are able to induce both Th1- and Th2-type immune responses, depending on the nature of the stimulation and the tissue microenvironment. As type-1 IFN was widely used as an antiviral agent and for the treatment of malignancies, clinicians naturally became interested in finding ways to manipulate the functioning of NIPCs in vivo.

During the 1990s, clinicians started to develop insights into the interactions of DCs with microbes, TAAs, autoantigens, allergens, and transplant antigens. Immunologists progressively developed better techniques for isolating DCs from various tissues, including human blood. Different investigators published their data on the induction and production of various cytokines, chemokines, and immune modulators, including type-1 IFN, by different subsets of DCs. Researchers of various disciplines started to work together, and by the late 1990s, DCs had begun to move from the lab bench to the bedside.

In addition to the DCs described above, there are some other cells with a dendritic morphology in the nervous system, but those are neither APCs nor related to the immune response.

Moreover, a third type of cells with dendritic morphology does participate in immune responses, although they are not professional APCs of the immune system. These cells are called follicular dendritic cells (FDCs) because they were first detected in the primary B-cell follicles of secondary lymphoid organs. FDCs share some morphological features with DCs, but they are otherwise quite different from the antigen-presenting DCs described above. FDCs can retain antigen—antibody complexes on their surfaces for long periods, but they cannot perform all the functions of professional APCs. Although the existence of these cells has been known since 1950, they were not characterized until 1962 or named until 1978. Between the early 1980s to the early 1990s, these cells were isolated and functionally evaluated.

The chronological history of immunology shows that we first came to know about antibodies "A" and their protective capacity two centuries ago. In the last century, we developed tremendous insights regarding the phenotypes, functions, and mechanism of action of T and B lymphocytes "B." During the middle of the 20th century, many cytokines "C," which are able to regulate different immune reactions, entered the immunological arena. In the final quarter of the last century, we achieved insights into APCs and DCs "D." Thus, it seems that the evolution of immunology has progressed in alphabetical order: A, B, C, and D. Now A, B, C, and D are meeting on the lab bench and at the bedside. Each discovery and innovation altered our understanding of the previous concepts tremendously. At this moment, we are unsure about "E" and its likely impact on its immediate predecessor D, dendritic cells.

Current Definition and Characteristics of Dendritic Cells

Several features of DCs, such as their ontogeny, phylogeny, and functions, are known. DCs can be isolated from different tissues, including peripheral blood, with more than 90% purity. However, a universal definition of DCs is not possible, mainly owing to the lack of a DC-specific marker, the presence of different subsets of DCs, and the rapid progress being made regarding the identification of new markers and functions of DCs. Only recently have DCs become accessible for detailed molecular and cell biological analyses. Microarray techniques and proteomics are emerging as potentially complementary technologies for identifying the mRNA and protein constituents of DCs. A global analysis of gene expression during DC differentiation and maturation has been started. The use of these technologies will make it possible to define DCs more precisely.

At present, DCs can be identified and functionally evaluated by using several characteristic features, as in the following list.

1. Many dendritic processes in some dendritic cells, especially following maturation and activation, very few in others
2. Versatile morphologically and functionally according to development, maturation, tissue of localization, and subsets
3. Sentinels in vivo: antigen-presenting functions include antigen capture and processing and migration to regional lymph nodes
4. Initiators of immune responses; stimulate quiescent, naive, and memory B and T lymphocytes
5. Strong potency in stimulating T lymphocytes: small numbers of dendritic cells and low levels of antigens induce strong T cell responses
6. Activation of natural killer (NK) cells and natural killer T (NKT) cells
7. Production of type-1 interferon by plasmacytoid dendritic cells.
8. Inducers of central and peripheral tolerance

Very few cells of the body are endowed with so many different phenotype or such diverse functional capabilities. The primary function of DCs is to act as sentinels of the immune system. Under steady-state conditions, DCs in the peripheral tissues recognize and process self-Ags, nondangerous stimuli, and other similar entities (Fig. 1.1). The outcome of these activities is the induction of immunogenic tolerance or unresponsiveness (Fig. 1.1A). This may be the principle function of DCs under normal physiological conditions. In contrast, when microbes, tumor cells, harmful entities, remains of necrotic cells, or apoptotic cells are present in the peripheral tissues, DCs may mobilize from the blood to the tissues. According to this scenario, these agents are then recognized by the interactions between pathogen-recognition receptors on DCs, such as Toll-like receptors, and their ligands on harmful entities (Fig. 1.1B). This leads to the capture, internalization, and processing of these agents by DCs (Fig 1.1C). Finally, DCs express Ag-peptides along with self-major histocompatibility complex (MHC) molecules. These DCs then become migratory, move to the lymphoid tissues, and enter into Ag-presentation mode (Fig. 1.1D). There, they activate lymphocytes at immunological synapses in the lymphoid tissues. All these cellular events lead to the production of Ag-specific T lymphocytes and B lymphocytes.

Concluding Remarks

Antigen-presenting DCs, like everything in science, are highly dynamic in nature. Several investigators around the world are working to learn about these cells. Many more markers and functions of DCs will be explored in the future. On the other hand, many features and functions that have been attributed to DCs will be challenged in

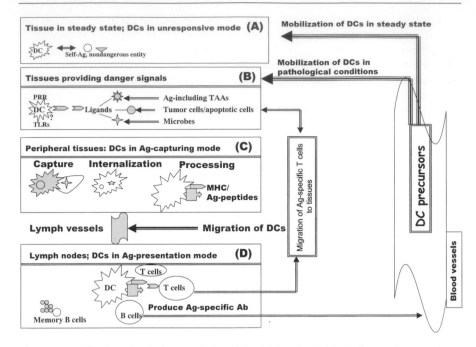

Fig. 1.1A–D. The functional characteristics of dendritic cells (*DCs*). In the steady state, tissue DCs induce immunological tolerance or unresponsiveness to *self-antigens* and possibly to *non-dangerous entities* (**A**). The putative functions of DCs in tissues receiving nonself-antigens or harmful signals are shown (**B–D**). When tumor-associated antigens (*TAAs*), *tumor cells*, *apoptotic cells*, or *microbes* are localized in the tissue, DC precursors might be mobilized from the blood. Immature DCs in the tissues would also recognize the pathogenic entities by their receptors (**B**). Mobilized DCs would capture, internalize, and process the pathogenic entities, and become activating DCs (**C**). These DCs would then migrate to the lymphoid tissues and activate the clonally selected lymphocytes (**D**). The products of these immunological responses are antigen-specific T and B lymphocytes. The antigen-specific T lymphocytes (*T cells*) might migrate to the tissue where the microbial invasion has occurred, whereas *B cells* produce antigen-specific antibodies. *Ag*, antigen; *PRR*, pattern-recognition receptor; *TLR*, toll-like receptor; *TAA*, tumor-associated antigen; *MHC*, major histocompatibility complex; *Ab*, antibody

the near future, and some may lose their validity. Whatever the situation might be, all these events will lead to the development of a proper understanding of DCs. In the first decade of the 21st century, we will gain a working understanding of the potential scope and limitations of DC applications as we gain insights into what DCs can and cannot do.

However, investigators should be cautious when applying the new information about DCs clinically. In general, clinicians pick up information from the lab bench and apply it at the bedside for the well-being of patients. Sometimes, this is done too hastily, without proper understanding of the conditions in situ. A period of chaos and confusion regarding aspects of DCs applied clinically could be avoided by establishing a scientific bridge between the basic investigator and the clinician.

Based on the experimental data, several trials of DC-based therapies or DC-targeting therapies for pathological conditions were initiated. However, many of these applied studies were based directly on understanding of pathological processes that was gained in animal models of human diseases. It is true that impaired functioning of DCs has been detected in patients with persistent infections, malignancies, and autoimmune and allergic diseases. However, functional impairment of DCs in pathological conditions might arise in two ways. The diseases might progress as a result of the defective functioning of DCs. Conversely, the pathological processes of various diseases might cause impaired functioning of DCs. Naturally, it is extremely hard to gain accurate insights into these cellular and molecular events in human beings.

Understanding the role of DCs in these pathological processes is important to determine whether a DC-based therapy might be beneficial. Currently, the trend is to administer Ag-pulsed DCs, activated DCs, or tolerogenic DCs to treat different pathological conditions without understanding the nature of the pathological processes or the role of DCs in vivo. The initial clinical trials of DC-based therapies have resulted in some encouraging outcomes. However, how many therapeutic trials did not achieve good outcomes and how many clinical trials ended with adverse outcomes? The reality of contemporary science seldom allows publication of negative or adverse data.

However, the true picture is not completely frustrating. The diverse origins, phenotypes, and functions of DCs imply that these unique cells have great potential for use in clinical situations. At the same time, it is dangerous for DCs to be brought to the bedside before an accurate understanding of their nature is obtained at the lab bench. The pathogenesis of the vast majority of diseases is still unknown. Different subsets of DCs might play divergent roles in pathological processes. Again, it is very important to gain accurate insights into the role of the disease microenvironment on the functioning of DCs, especially in long-lasting pathological processes in vivo. Finally, biologists who study DCs should evaluate the scope and limitations of DC-based therapies on a case-by-case basis so that this promising approach does not end up being abandoned, as has happened with many other apparently promising immune therapies previously.

Recommended Readings

Banchereau J, Steinman RM (1998) Dendritic cells and the control of immunity. Nature 392:245–252

Banchereau J, Briere F, Caux C, et al. (1999) Immunobiology of dendritic cells. Annu Rev Immunol 18:767–818

Langerhans P (1868) Über die nerven der menschlichen haut. Virchows Arch (Pathol Anat) 44:323–327

Steinman RM (1991) The dendritic cell system and its role in immunogenicity. Annu Rev Immunol 9:271–296

Steinman RM, Cohn ZA (1973) Identification of a novel cell type in peripheral lymphoid organs of mice. I. Morphology, quantitation, tissue distribution. J Exp Med 137:1142–1162

Tew JG, Wu J, Qin D, et al. (1997) Follicular dendritic cells and presentation of antigen and costimulatory signals to B cells. Immunol Rev 156:39–52

2. General Features of Dendritic Cells

Outline

General Considerations

The most rapidly evolving aspect of dendritic cell (DC) biology is the magnificent diversity of phenotypes that have been described from both mice and humans through in vitro and in vivo studies. Initially, DCs were defined as a trace population of immunocytes that were negative for markers of myeloid and lymphoid lineages and expressed very high levels of major histocompatibility complex (MHC) class II antigens, a hallmark of antigen-presenting cells (APCs). Functionally, DCs were found to be potent stimulators of allogenic T cells in vitro. Phase contrast microscopy revealed the existence of dendritic processes on DCs. Many new features of DCs have since been discovered, and several characteristics previously attributed to DCs are no longer considered valid.

At present, DCs, possibly in different forms or with different phenotypes, can be detected or isolated from most lymphoid and nonlymphoid organs. They are highly divergent with respect to their level of maturation and functioning. Furthermore, DCs having different forms and functions may be present in a single tissue. Thus, the most important problem is to properly define DCs. The problem is further accentuated because most of the different types of DCs observed in vivo have been defined by their functional characteristics. DC progenitors represent a population of hematopoietic stem cells that become DCs when they receive the requisite signals in vivo or the appropriate cytokines in vitro. These DC progenitor cells are positive for cluster of differentiation 34 (CD34$^+$) and retain the potential to proliferate. DC precursors, which are more committed than DC progenitors to become DCs, are generated from DC progenitors. The features of the progenitor and precursor cells of most DC subsets have not been defined, except for human plasmacytoid DCs. Some DC precursors, such as monocytes, are highly differentiated, whereas the phenotypes of other DC precursors have not yet been described. Immature DCs, which are mainly present in nonlymphoid tissues, are the sentinels of the immune system. Their major functions include recognition and capture of antigens (Ags) and apoptotic cells. They express low levels of costimulatory molecules. Maturing and migratory DCs represent a population of DCs that have engulfed and processed Ags. They also show altered chemokine receptor expression. Mature DCs are usually formed in the lymphoid tissues during their interaction with lymphocytes; however, they are also found in nonlymphoid tissues, especially in diseased tissues. Tolerogenic DCs induce immune tolerance either because of their low expression of costimulatory molecules or by their production of inhibitory cytokines or mediators. After a period of stimulation, DCs sometimes reach a state of exhaustion. Killer DCs express Fas ligand (FasL) and might kill target cells, but the capacity of killer DCs to destroy target cells in vivo is not well documented. Although different types of DCs are described here, their extreme plasticity and diversity do not allow these DCs to be properly identified in situ.

Limitations of Defining DCs by Dendritic Morphology

The name *dendritic cell* implies that, morphologically, these cells have dendritic processes; however, DCs from most tissues and organs do not show such processes. Freshly isolated DCs seldom exhibit their dendritic processes, and some DCs actually do not have any dendritic processes of note. In others, the dendritic processes can be detected only in some maturational phases and activation states.

Defining DCs in a particular tissue by the presence of dendritic processes is also impossible. Several types of DCs, including DC progenitors, DC precursors, immature DCs, maturing DCs, mature DCs, tolerogenic DCs, exhausted DCs, and killer DCs, might be present in the same organ or tissue at the same time, and only a few of these DCs might show dendritic processes.

When DCs are isolated from different tissues, whether dendritic processes are observed depends on the duration of the culture, the presence of cytokines in the culture, and the type of DC being cultured.

Limitations of Defining DCs by Surface Markers

When a cell cannot be defined by morphology, an alternative way to identify that cell in different tissues and organs is by its immunohistochemistry or flow cytometry. To identify cells by these techniques, cell-specific markers must be expressed in those cells but not in adjacent cells or in contaminated cell populations.

DCs were originally thought to be negative for lineage markers (markers for cells of myeloid or lymphoid lineage). However, it is now becoming evident that some antigens associated with myeloid and lymphoid lineages are constitutively expressed by different subsets of DCs. Moreover, several markers for myeloid and lymphoid cells can also be detected on DCs in vitro, depending on the culture conditions. Although DCs, like most immunocytes, express several APC-related antigens (MHC class II, CD80, CD86, CD40, and CD54) on their surface, none is DC-specific. Many of these markers can be detected on cells that are localized adjacent to DCs in vivo and in cells that contaminate DCs in culture.

Most importantly, no marker is expressed on different subsets of DCs. Also, the DC phenotype varies considerably depending on its stage of activation or maturation.

Phenotypic Diversity of DCs

DCs can thus be defined neither by their dendritic morphology nor by the expression of DC-specific surface antigens. It is possible, however, to understand the causes underlying the phenotypic diversity of DCs. First, we need to look at the historical events relating to the discovery of DCs and their phenotypic characterization. DCs were first isolated from murine spleen by over-night culture of spleen cells. The spleen is a secondary lymphoid organ, and many of the isolated spleen DCs would have been likely to have encountered microbial agents, their antigens, or other cellular sources of antigens. Some of the isolated DCs might have migrated from the peripheral tissues. These DCs would not have been in antigen-capture mode, but instead would have been assigned to interact with T lymphocytes in the spleen. Naturally, most exhibited a comparatively mature phenotype. Moreover, because they were isolated by overnight culture of spleen cells, they had a further opportunity to undergo maturation during culture. The matured phenotype of the isolated spleen DCs was also reflected in their functional capacities. Very few were able to stimulate allogenic T cells in an allogenic mixed leukocyte reaction. Bulk populations of spleen DCs were also potent inducers and producers of various inflammatory cytokines and immune mediators. However, when fresh spleen DCs were enriched by cell sorting techniques, comparatively fewer mature DCs were isolated. In general, both immature and mature DCs were found among spleen DCs.

The DC phenotypes present in a tissue depend on the tissue microenvironment. Although both spleen and thymus are lymphoid organs, DCs in the thymus may perform a very specialized job. Accordingly, the phenotypes of thymic DCs differ considerably from those of DCs of the spleen and other lymphoid organs.

When DCs were localized in or isolated from nonlymphoid tissues, a completely different picture emerged. DCs could not be identified in many nonlymphoid tissues by using known DC-specific markers; in fact, very few DCs could be identified in most of these tissues. This is not surprising because probably very few DCs in nonlymphoid tissues are resting. DCs reach the nonlymphoid tissues through circulation. Naturally, most of these DCs have an immature phenotype because their function is to capture microbes or their antigens or apoptotic cells. In the steady state, antigen uptake by these DCs leads to immune tolerance, which under physiological conditions may be the main role of DCs. When there is a danger signal or inflammatory stimulus in peripheral tissues, some of these DCs capture antigens and undergo partial maturation. These maturing DCs may leave the nonlymphoid tissue and migrate to lymphoid tissues. Accordingly, DC phenotypes in nonlymphoid tissues are diverse and depend on the nature of the organ.

Figure 2.1 is a schema showing a possible life history of DCs and the tissues of localization associated with each maturational state. It is evident that DCs with different phenotypes and functions, such as DC progenitors, DC precursors, immature DCs, maturing DCs, migrating DCs, and mature DCs can be localized in most lymphoid and nonlymphoid tissues. However, it is not clear whether there are organ-specific DCs. Insights into this problem await the discovery of tissue-specific DC progenitors in some organs.

Ideally, DC progenitors should be studied in detail before DCs. However, this progression did not occur for historical reasons. DC phenotypes could not be investigated methodically as would be scientifically ideal; instead, they were studied in the order that they were isolated from different tissues and as various DC-related Ags became available. It is well known that DCs, including those from spleen, are bone marrow-derived, where they are generated from $CD34^+$ hematopoietic progenitor cells (HPCs). However, DC progenitors [precursors] were not isolated until more than

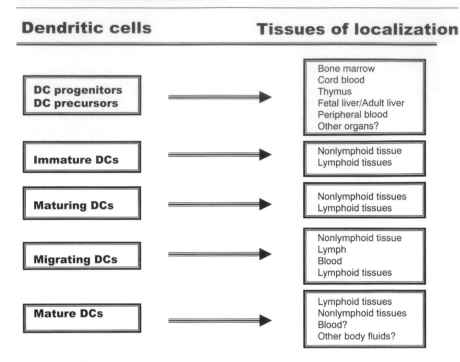

Fig. 2.1. The life history of dendritic cells (DCs) and their tissues of localization. DCs with different maturational and functional states can be detected from a variety of organs. The *progenitors* and *precursors* of DCS are found in the *bone marrow, blood,* and *thymus,* and in peripheral tissues. *Immature, maturing, migrating,* and *mature* DCs have been localized from both *nonlymphoid* and *lymphoid tissues*

a decade after the isolation of spleen DCs. In fact, we are only now learning about DC progenitors and precursors, more than two decades after the first discovery of their mature counterparts (spleen DCs).

Factors Complicating the Characterization of Dendritic Cells

The morphology of DCs varies considerably depending on their tissue of localization, their level of maturation, and their degree of activation. Moreover, there is no universal DC-specific marker capable of identifying DCs from various tissues. This situation complicates the phenotyping of DCs from different tissues and organs, but some new information has made the picture even more confusing. Initially, DCs were thought to be lineage negative: they did not express markers for lymphoid or myeloid lineages. However, it was eventually found that DCs from some tissues do express some markers for myeloid and lymphoid lineages. Moreover, although DCs were long thought to be negative for Fc receptors, it is now apparent that DCs from several sources do express them. This new information is highly important for the characterization of DCs and for designing DC-based therapies, but it makes the identification of DCs difficult.

Concluding Remarks

It is evident that it is extremely difficult to define DCs properly. However, a working definition of DCs based on current knowledge about these cells is needed. DCs belong to the common leukocyte family, and all DCs express the marker for the common leukocyte lineage. DCs do not express T-cell markers such as CD3, but some DCs express other T-cell differentiation markers such as CD4 and CD8. Murine, but not human, DCs, express some B-cell markers. Monocytes and macrophages share many common markers with DCs. These types of cells may also convert into DCs both in vivo and in vitro. Functionally, the only characteristic that is unique to DCs is their capacity to induce the proliferation and polarization of naive T cells. All other functions of DCs can be performed by other cells, although DCs perform these functions with greater efficiency. A working definition of DCs might thus be derived from their phenotypic and functional characteristics. DCs are a trace population of immunocytes with certain properties. They (1) express dendritic processes and some markers suggestive of their phylogeny and phenotype; (2) are capable of capturing, recognizing, and processing antigens, microbial agents, tumor cells, and apoptotic cells; (3) are able to migrate; and (4) possess the ability to interact with T lymphocytes efficiently.

Phenotypes of Dendritic Cells

DC Phenotypes from Lymphoid Tissues

DCs are derived from bone marrow, and they become localized to lymphoid tissues after migration from the bone marrow via the blood. The signals that induce the migration of DCs from the bone marrow to different lymphoid tissues remain to be elucidated. On the other hand, the bulk of DCs in the lymphoid tissues may come from nonlymphoid tissues after encountering microbes or Ags or owing to the influence of inflammatory stimuli. Thus, DCs with different states of maturation and activation may be found in the lymphoid tissues.

DCs are detectable in the lymphoid tissues of different animals, including humans. However, DCs from murine lymphoid tissues have been most extensively studied because huge numbers of DCs can be isolated from these tissues. Moreover, lymphoid tissue-derived DCs have been used for DC-based therapies in mice.

DCs in Murine Spleen and Lymph Nodes

DCs in the murine spleen were first identified by their expression of antigens that reacted with the rat monoclonal antibody (mAb) 33D1. However, detailed studies on the localization and functional characteristics of 33D1$^+$ spleen DCs have not been carried out. Most importantly, details of the structure of this antigen and biochemical data regarding 33D1 are not available. 33D1 is no longer used to define spleen DC phenotypes.

A summary of DC phenotypes in murine lymphoid tissues is shown in Table 2.1. DCs in murine lymphoid tissues are best characterized by their expression of antigens such as CD11c, DEC-205, and CD8α.

Table 2.1. Phenotypes of DCs in murine lymphoid tissues. In mice, CD11c is a common marker of DCs. In murine lymphoid tissues, different subtypes of DCs are distinguished by their expression of *CD8α*. *Plasmacytoid* DCs are identified by their expression of *B220* and *Gr-1*. *Thymic DCs express BP-1*

Tissue	Dendritic cells	Phenotypes
Spleen	Lymphoid	$CD11c^+$, $CD8\alpha^+$, DEC-205$^+$, $CD11b^{-/nil}$
	Myeloid	$CD11c^+$, $CD8\alpha^-$, DEC-205$^-$, $CD11b^+$
	Plasmacytoid	$CD11c^{low}$, $CD11b^-$, $CD45RA^{high}$
		$CD11c^+$, $B220^+$, $CD11b^-$, $Gr-1^+$
Lymph node	Lymphoid	$CD11c^+$, $CD8\alpha^+$, DEC-205$^+$, $CD11b^{-/nil}$
	Myeloid	$CD11c^+$, $CD8\alpha^-$, DEC-205$^-$, $CD11b^+$
	Plasmacytoid	$CD11c^{low}$, $CD11b^-$, $CD45RA^{high}$
		$CD11c^+$, $B220^+$, $CD11b^-$, $Gr-1^+$
Thymic DCs		$CD11c^+$, DEC-205$^+$, $CD8\alpha^+$, $BP-1^+$
Peyer's patch	T-cell area	$CD11c^+$, DEC-205$^+$, $CD8\alpha^+$
	Subdome	$CD11c^+$, DEC-205$^-$, $CD8\alpha^-$

Rat mAb N418 binds a CD11c epitope and is expressed at high density on DCs from most murine lymphoid tissues. Another antibody (Ab), DEC-205, reacts with rat mAb nonlymphoid dendritic cell (NLDC) 145. The rat NLDC-145 mAb was raised by immunizing a rat with mouse lymphoid-tissue sarcoma and screening for reactivity to DCs in tissue sections. Subsequent isolation of an Ag recognized by NLDC-145 and protein sequencing enabled a full-length mouse cDNA to be isolated. NLDC-145 was renamed as DEC-205 after its molecular weight was revised. DEC-205 has some similarity to macrophage mannose receptor. Although both DEC-205 and CD11c are widely expressed on mouse lymphoid DCs, they are not DC-specific because DEC-205 is also expressed on macrophages, and CD11c is also detected on other leukocytes, including macrophages.

Based on the expression of these antigens, the following subsets of DCs have been identified in murine lymphoid tissues (spleen and lymph nodes).

Putative Lymphoid-Related DCs or $CD8\alpha^+$ DCs. Phenotypically, the lymphoid-related DCs are $CD11c^+$, $CD8\alpha^+$, DEC-205$^+$, $CD11b^{-/nil}$. They are present in both spleen and lymph nodes. In the spleen, $CD8\alpha^+$ DCs are localized deep in the T-cell-rich areas of the periarteriolar lymphatic sheaths (PALS). A similar distribution of $CD8\alpha^+$ DCs is seen in the lymph nodes.

Putative Myeloid DCs or $CD8\alpha^-$ DCs. Myeloid DCs have the phenotype $CD11c^+$, DEC-205$^-$, $CD8\alpha^-$. They are present in both spleen and lymph nodes. In the spleen, they are localized to the marginal zone. However, activation of these DCs by lipopolysaccharide or toxoplasma extracts induces their migration from the marginal zone to the T-cell-rich PALS. In the lymph nodes, these DCs reside mostly in the subcapsular sinus, and in the PALS region, adjacent to the B-cell follicles.

Langerhans Cell DCs. A subset of DCs with the phenotype $CD11c^+$, $CD8\alpha^{+/-}$, DEC-205$^+$ is present in murine spleen. In culture, these DCs can acquire the Langerhans cell (LC) phenotype. They are detected in the lymph nodes but not in the spleen.

Although these three DC subsets in the lymphoid tissues show strikingly different phenotypes, they express similar levels of molecules involved with antigen presentation, such as MHC class II, CD40, CD80, and CD86.

Type-1 Interferon-Producing DCs or Plasmacytoid DCs. In addition to these three DC phenotypes, a population of CD11c$^+$ DCs expressing B220 and Gr-1 antigens has recently been detected from the murine spleen and lymph nodes. Another recent study found CD11c^{low}, CD11b$^-$, CD45RA^{high} DCs in the spleen. These DCs may be equivalent to the plasmacytoid DCs, or natural interferon-producing cells (NIPCs), of human peripheral blood, and they produce abundant amounts of type-1 interferon (IFN) in vitro in response to viral infection. However, in contrast to human plasmacytoid DCs, they are CD11c$^+$. Moreover, a dependency of murine type-1 IFN-producing DCs on interleukin (IL)-3 has not been clearly shown.

Phenotypes of DCs in Human Spleen, Lymph Nodes, and Tonsils

Different types of DCs and DC-like cells have been identified in human spleen and lymph nodes by immunohistochemistry. These cells can be detected in different compartments of the human spleen: in the T-cell-rich areas of the PALS, in the B-cell-rich follicles, and in the intrafollicular mantle. As both DCs and macrophages are seen in these compartments, and there are no DC-specific markers in humans, it is unclear which of these cells are true DCs. Extensive studies to define DC phenotypes in human spleen and lymph nodes have not been carried out.

In humans, at least three subsets of DCs have been characterized in the tonsils: numbers 1 and 2, below, are in the PALS and the number 3 is in the B-cell-rich follicles.

1. Interdigitating DCs expressing CD11c, CD40, CD86, and CD83 have been detected in T-cell-rich areas of the tonsils. DCs with different states of maturation can be further subdivided by their expression of CD83.
2. CD4$^+$, CD3$^-$, CD11c$^-$ DCs are present in T-cell-rich areas and around the high endothelial venules of tonsils. The precursors of these cells are also found in the blood. Cells with this phenotype are known as plasmacytoid T cells, plasmacytoid DCs, or NIPCs.
3. CD4$^+$, CD11c$^+$, CD3$^-$ DCs found in the germinal center of the tonsils are known as germinal center DCs (GCDCs). GCDCs express Fcγ receptors such as CD16, CD32, and CD64. GCDCs represent the mature progeny of CD11c$^+$ DC precursors in the blood.

Recently, tonsillar DCs both in situ and from isolated tonsillar cells were broadly classified into five subsets based on their expression of HLA DR, CD11c, and CD123: (1) HLA DR^{mod}, CD11c$^-$, CD123$^+$; (2) HLA DR^{high}, CD11c$^-$, CRMF44^{high}; (3) HLA DR^{mod}, CD11c$^-$, CD13$^-$, CRMF44^{low}; (4) HLA DR^{mod}, CD11c$^-$, CD123$^-$; and (5) HLA DR^{mod}, CD11c$^+$ germinal center DC. The functional implications of these subsets and their compartmentalization in the tonsils have not been defined.

Thymic DCs in Mice and Humans

Thymic DCs in mice originate from thymic precursors and are more closely related to lymphocytes than to cells of myeloid origin. Freshly isolated thymic DCs do not show a dendritic morphology, and they express dendritic processes only after long culture. Murine thymic DCs are MHC class I$^+$, MHC class II$^+$, CD11c$^+$, DEC-205$^+$, CD8α$^+$, CD11b$^{dull/-}$, CD86$^+$, and CD40$^+$. The thymic DC phenotype is very similar to that of a DC subset of the spleen and lymph node. One marker that is not expressed by spleen or lymph node DCs but is expressed by thymic DCs is BP-1, a glutamyl aminopeptidase. This is an early B-cell marker. BP-I is produced by DCs because it is not washed out during culture. Some thymic DCs express FasL, Thy 1.1, and Thy 1.2. These molecules may result from the tight junction with T cells and are lost during culture. A subset of thymic DCs also expresses CD25.

CD34$^+$ CD38^{dim} thymic precursors in humans can be differentiated in the presence of granulocyte-macrophage colony-stimulating factor (GM-CSF) and tumor necrosis factor (TNF)-α into T lymphocytes, natural killer (NK) cells, and DCs. In humans, three distinct populations of thymic DCs have been identified: (1) CD11c$^+$, CD11b$^-$, CD45RO^{low} DCs do not express myeloid markers and can be induced to produce IL-12; (2) CD11c^{high}, CD11b$^+$, CD45RO^{high} DCs constitute a minor population and are weak producers of IL-12; and (3) CD11c$^-$, CD123$^+$, which does not produce IL-12. Human thymic DCs do not express CD8.

DCs in Peyer's Patch

Peyer's patch (PP) is the main lymphoid organ where Ags are made available to the immune cells of the gut. Ags may be transported to PP by specialized gut cells called M cells. DCs have been described in two PP sites: T-cell areas and the subepithelial area underlying the dome. In general, DCs in the gut express CD11c. Subdome DCs are negative for DEC-205, but those in the T-cell areas express DEC-205. Subdome DCs express a typical marker of myeloid DCs, CD11b, whereas DCs in T-cell areas express CD8α, a lymphoid DC marker. A third DC population that is CD11c$^+$ but negative for CD11b and DEC-205 is also found in the gut. Little is known about DCs in PP in humans.

DCs in Cryptopatches

In addition to PP, the gut has solitary lymphoid structures that may be sites of extrathymic T-cell differentiation. In mice, these structures are called cryptopatches, and cryptopatch-like structures have also been detected in rats. Moreover, structures resembling cryptopatches have also been described in the human small intestine. MHC class II-positive DCs have been detected in the cryptopatch-like structures in human small intestine along with memory T cells and a variable B-cell component.

Summary of DCs in Lymphoid Tissues

DCs with different phenotypes are present in all lymphoid tissues in both humans and mice. For example, DCs in the PALS T-cell region of the spleen are CD11c$^+$, DEC-205$^+$, and CD8α$^+$, whereas those in the marginal zone do not express DEC-205 or CD8α. What is the significance of this phenotypic heterogeneity? Is it determined during development? DCs in the lymphoid tissues presumably come from nonlymphoid tissues after encountering antigens, or they may migrate to the lymphoid tissues directly from the bone marrow. Whether the compartmentalization of different subtypes of DCs to the PALS or the marginal zone of the spleen is dependent on the nature of the stimuli received at the periphery is an open question. It is also possible that terminally differentiated DCs are localized in different compartments of the lymphoid tissues by the influence of chemokines or other stimuli.

Plasmacytoid DCs have been isolated from the spleen and the lymph nodes, but the site of their localization in lymphoid tissues is not known except in tonsils.

To date, bulk populations of DCs from lymphoid tissues have been used for immune therapy, especially in the mouse model. It is now evident that there are both putative immunogenic and tolerogenic DCs among the bulk population of DCs. For example, murine lymphoid DCs expressing $CD8\alpha$ produce IL-12. More understanding about the relationship between DC phenotypic diversity and function is needed to put the use of DCs in therapy on a more rational basis.

Phenotypes of Dendritic Cells in Nonlymphoid Tissues

DCs have been enriched or isolated from most tissues of the body except the nervous system. Nonlymphoid tissues contain different types of DCs with diverse phenotypes and functions. In some tissues, DCs have been localized immunohistochemically, whereas in others DCs have been propagated in vitro by culturing precursor populations in the presence of various cytokines. Thus, it is hard to define the nature and phenotype of DCs in situ in different nonlymphoid tissues because their phenotypes might be altered during in vitro culture.

DCs in the Skin (Langerhans Cells)

Langerhans cells (LCs) reside mainly within the stratified squamous epithelia, where they compose 2%–4% of all epithelial cells. In the epidermis, LCs are located in the suprabasal position and remain attached to neighboring keratinocytes via an E-cadherin- and Ca^{2+}-dependent mechanism. LC density varies from location to location. One study showed that there were about 200 LCs/mm^2 in the palm and about 930 LCs/mm^2 in the epidermis of the face and neck.

LCs are characterized by the presence of Birbeck granules. Resident LCs display nonspecific esterase and ATPase activity. They also express Fc-immunoglobulin (Ig) G type II receptors (FCγRII, CD32), an Fc-IgE type I receptor (FCεR1), and C3bi receptors (CD11b–CD18). LCs also express langerin in the membrane.

Although specific markers for human or mouse LCs are lacking, in general, molecules such as CD11c, MHC class II, and DEC-205 indicate mouse LCs, and others such as CD1a and CD1c are used to describe human LCs. Recently, an antibody has been discovered that identifies langerin, a 40-kDa LC molecule. This antibody is called DCGM4. Langerin is a type II Ca^{2+}-dependent lectin displaying mannose-binding specificity that co-localizes with Birbeck granules. Langerin may be an antigen-capturing apparatus that channels antigens to the Birbeck granules, but this has not been confirmed.

The murine LC phenotype depends on their level of maturation or activation. Resting LCs are identified by their expression of CD11c, langerin, E-cadherin, and low costimulatory molecules. On the other hand, activated LCs express very high levels of activation and maturation markers. These markers include CD80 and CD86.

In humans, two subsets of LCs can be distinguished by their expression of HLA DR: HLA DR^{low} and HLA DR^{high}. These subsets may reflect the maturational state.

In addition to LCs, another type of DCs in the skin is called dermal dendritic cells (DDCs). In mice, two populations of DDCs have been described: CD11b$^+$ and CD11b$^-$. DDCs express most of the molecules that mature LCs express, but they also express intracytoplasmic transglutaminase clotting factor VIIIa (FXVIIIa), CD1b, and lower levels of CD1a and CD1c than LCs. DDCs can be distinguished from LCs by the absence of E-cadherin or langerin expression.

DCs in the Lung, Gut, Liver, Kidney, Heart, and Pancreas

Lung. In the lung, DCs are found in the bronchial mucosa either above or below the basement membrane, or deep in the lamina propria of the bronchia. DCs are also seen in the bronchial-associated lymphoid tissue in the mucosa below the epithelium. Many DCs are found in the perivascular lymphoid tissue and the pleura. Lung DCs are immature and very similar to freshly isolated blood DCs. One major problem regarding phenotyping of lung DCs is that CD11c is expressed on both DCs and monocytes of the lung. Lung DCs express high levels of MHC class II molecules, lymphocyte function-associated (LFA)-3 antigens, and low levels of CD14. Lung DCs, like other immature DCs, express very low levels of CD86, CD80, and CD40, and they do not express CD1a. CD83 is almost nonexistent on lung DCs, again indicating that these DCs are immature.

Gut. From data of immunohistochemical, immunofluorescence, and morphological studies, it is apparent that DCs are abundant in the gut. The majority lie in the lamina propria (LP), underlying the epithelia. However, recent evidence suggests that DCs may extend their processes above the basement membrane. The projection of dendritic processes above the basement membrane under physiological conditions has not been shown. However, following infection with *Salmonella typhimurium,* DCs in the gut are able to send dendritic processes outside the gut epithelium. DCs are also able to open the tight junction between the epithelial cells and directly sample microbes in the gut lumen. As DCs contain tight-junction proteins such as occludin, claudin 1, and zonula occludens 1, the integrity of the epithelial barrier is preserved even after the dendritic processes periscope out. Adequate phenotypic studies of human gut DCs have not been done. Immunohistochemical studies of the human gut have detected both immature and mature DCs.

Liver. Murine liver harbors at least two populations of DCs, although their phenotypic and functional interrelationship is unclear. Liver DC progenitors can be propagated by culturing a progenitor population in hepatic nonparenchymal cells (NPCs) with GM-CSF for 7 days. A highly immature population of DC progenitors that does not undergo maturation and activation in the presence of proinflammatory cytokines such as IFN-γ and TNF-α was enriched for a functional study. However, these putative DC progenitors underwent maturation in the presence of intracellular matrix. It is thus elusive whether liver DC progenitors arise from a committed DC precursor or from other hematopoietic stem cells. These cells have never been localized in vivo.

CD11c$^+$ DCs are also located in the liver, mainly at the portal and along the central vein. Few CD11c$^+$ DCs are seen in the hepatic parenchyma. These DCs display all of the phenotypic features of DCs and are potent stimulators of allogenic T lymphocytes.

Treatment of mice with GM-CSF induces a population of DEC-205$^+$ DCs in the liver. There are four subsets of freshly isolated liver DCs based on the expression of B220, CD4, and CD11b: (1) CD11c$^+$, B220$^+$, CD4$^+$; (2) CD11c$^+$, B220$^+$, CD4$^-$; (3) CD11c$^+$, B220$^-$, CD11b$^+$; and (4) CD11c$^+$, B220$^-$, CD11b$^-$. Subsets 1 and 2 resemble plasmacytoid DCs, except for being Gr-1$^-$. In another study in which liver DCs were propagated by fms-like tyrosine kinase receptor 3 ligand (Flt-3L), two subsets of liver DCs were detected by their mutually exclusive expression of CD11b and CD8α.

Very few studies have been undertaken on the phenotypes of DCs in the human liver, especially in the physiological liver. A flow cytometric study showed that liver-derived DCs express CD11c and CD123, but contamination from blood could not be completely ruled out. Mature DCs expressing CD83 have been detected in the liver, especially under pathological conditions.

Kidney, Heart, and Pancreas. Immunohistochemical studies have identified DCs in the kidney, heart, and pancreas, but extensive phenotypic characterization of DCs from these organs has not been done.

Summary of DCs in the Nonlymphoid Tissues

DCs have been found in most nonlymphoid tissues, but a proper phenotypic characterization has not been done. In general, nonlymphoid tissue DCs are immature and their function is to capture antigens. However, mature DCs expressing maturation and activation markers have been found in many tissues. It is unclear how mature DCs are localized in these tissues; many nonlymphoid organs also have some lymphoid tissues. It is still unknown whether immature DCs in nonlymphoid tissues present antigens to the lymphoid tissues of the same organs. This may be especially important under pathological conditions.

Phenotypes of DCs from Human Peripheral Blood

Murine spleen- and lymph node-derived DCs are extensively used to study DCs, but human DCs cannot easily be studied because human spleen and lymph node are not readily available. Although it is not clear whether both immature and mature DCs are present in human peripheral blood, there is ample evidence suggesting that DC progenitors and precursors are present. DCs, along with other cells of the hematopoietic system, originate from CD34$^+$ HPCs, which have been detected in peripheral blood, cord blood, and fetal liver. The phenotypes of DC progenitors and precursors in human peripheral blood are summarized in Fig. 2.2.

Subsets of Peripheral Blood DCs (PBDCs) Based on the Expression of CD11c

Precursor populations of DCs originated from CD34$^+$ HPCs have been identified and characterized from human peripheral blood. Two main DC precursors in peripheral blood have been identified based on their expression of CD11c and CD123: CD11C$^+$, CD123$^{-/low}$ and CD11c$^-$, CD123$^+$. Both of these subsets are HLA DR$^+$ and negative for CD13.

CD11c$^+$ DC precursors undergo maturation in the presence of GM-CSF in vitro. They exhibit a myeloid appearance, and are regarded as myeloid DCs. On the other

DC progenitors
CD34⁺, CD33⁺ Myeloid progenitors
CD34⁺, CD10⁺ Lymphoid progenitors
Early progenitors of PDCs CD34⁺, CD4⁺, CD123⁺, CD45RA⁻
Late progenitors of PDCs CD34⁺, CD4⁺, CD123⁺, CD45RA⁺

DC precursors

Myeloid precursors:
Monocytes/CD14+
Lin-, CD11C⁺, CD13⁺, CD33⁺, CD14⁺
Lin-, CD11c⁺, CD13⁺, CD33⁺, CD14⁻
Lin-, CD11c⁺, CD123⁻, CD4⁺
Lin-, CD11c⁺, ILT-3⁺, ILT-1⁺, CD13⁺, CD33⁺

Lymphoid precursors:
Lin⁻, CD11c⁻, CD123⁺, CD4⁺
Lin⁻, CD11c⁻, ILT-1⁻, ILT-3⁺

Intermediate precursors of PDCs
CD34⁺, CD45RA⁺⁺, CD4⁺⁺, CD123⁺⁺

DC precursors based on CD1a expression
CD11c⁺, CD1a⁺, CD13⁺, CD33⁺
CD11c⁺, CD1a⁻, CD13⁺, CD33⁺

DC precursors based on BDCA expression
CD11c⁺, CD123⁻ [BDCA-3]
CD11c⁻, CD123⁺ [BDCA-2, 4]

Fig. 2.2. *Progenitors* and *precursors* of DCs are detected in human peripheral blood. DC progenitors are *CD34⁺*, and they can be divided into early and late progenitors. All DC precursors are lineage⁻, but they express CD4 antigen. Various *myeloid* and *lymphoid* markers are used to define myeloid and lymphoid precursors. Different subtypes of blood dentritic cells may be defined by the expression of blood dendritic cell antigens (BDCAs). *PDC*, plasmacytoid dendritic cell

hand, CD11c⁻ DC precursors undergo maturation in the presence of IL-3 and possess a lymphoid appearance; these cells are regarded as plasmacytoid DCs. They express only low levels of adhesion and costimulatory molecules such as CD80, CD86, and CD40, suggesting that they are relatively immature. CD83 is also not expressed on DC precursors in peripheral blood. However, when these DC precursors are cultured in vitro with inflammatory stimuli, they express high levels of adhesion and costimulatory molecules, depending on the culture conditions. Although these DC precursors become DCs during in vitro culture, there is no definitive proof that such an event takes place in vivo, especially in peripheral blood. However, these precursor populations of DCs might migrate to other tissues in response to inflammatory or danger signals. Their differentiation in other tissues has not been studied in detail, but the tissue microenvironment would influence further differentiation.

PBDCs That Express Neither CD11c nor CD123

In addition to the presence of precursors of myeloid and plasmacytoid DCs, another population of DC precursors in peripheral blood is lin⁻, HLA DR⁺, CD11c⁻, and CD123⁻.

Subset of DCs Based on the Expression of CD1a

Although CD1a is known to be expressed on human LCs, PBDCs can be divided into three subsets based on their expression of CD11c and CD1a. Two of these subsets belong to CD11c$^+$ DCs of the myeloid lineage: CD11c$^+$, CD1a$^+$ and CD11c$^+$, CD1a$^-$. Both CD11c$^+$ fractions display myeloid markers such as CD13 and CD33 and possess a GM-CSF receptor. When cultured in vitro, CD11c$^+$, CD1a$^+$ DCs took on the morphology of LCs and expressed langerin and E-cadherin and produced typical Birbeck granules. However, CD11c$^+$ CD1a$^-$ did not develop any LC characteristics under any culture conditions. The third subset of DCs in the blood is negative for both CD11c and CD1a and possibly belongs to the CD11c$^-$ plasmacytoid DCs.

Subsets of PBDCs Based on the Expression of Blood Dendritic Cell Antigen

An antigen that is specifically expressed on all types of DCs is lacking. However, some investigators have developed antibodies that react with some antigens on peripheral blood DCs. These antigens are called blood dendritic cell antigens (BDCAs), and panels of antibodies that identify antigens on different PBDC subsets are called anti-BDCAs. There are four BDCAs. Of these, three react with different types of DC in peripheral blood; BDCA-2 and BDCA-4 are detected on precursors of Plamacytoid DCs (CD11c$^-$, CD123$^+$ subset of PBDCs), and BDCA-3 binds to precursors of myeloid DCs in peripheral blood (CD11c$^+$, CD123$^-$ subset).

Blood DC Subset Based on the Expression of Immunoglobulin-like Transcript

Immunoglobulin-like transcript (ILT) is a novel molecule that was cloned from Epstein-Barr virus cell lines. Two types of ILTs, ILT1 and ILT3, are relevant to the phenotypic characterization of blood DCs. Myeloid blood DCs are CD11c$^+$, ILT3$^+$, ILT1$^+$, CD13$^+$, CD33$^+$, whereas plasmacytoid DCs are CD11c$^-$, CD123$^+$, ILT-1$^-$, ILT3$^+$. Both of these subsets express CD4, cutaneous leukocyte antigen (CLA), E-cadherin, CD40, CD86, and CD80, but only the ILT3$^+$ subset expresses CD62L and CXCR3.

Phenotypes of Cultured Blood DCs

Although different population of DCs can be derived by culturing DC precursors identified by their expression of CD11c, CD123, CD1, and ILTs, DCs can be also be produced by culturing monocytes or an adherent population of peripheral blood mononuclear cells (PBMCs) with GM-CSF and IL-4 for 7 days. These cultured DCs express HLA DR and CD11c, low to moderate levels of costimulatory antigens such as CD86 and CD80, and only very low levels of CD83. These DCs are inherently immature, but maturation can be induced by further culture with some inflammatory cytokines. A population of monocyte-derived DCs expresses DC-specific intracellular adhesion molecule 3 (ICAM-3)-grabbing nonintegrin (DC-SIGN). DC-SIGN has been reported to bind with human immunodeficiency virus (HIV) 1, but its implications regarding monocyte-derived DCs are as yet unknown. DC-SIGN is not expressed on plasmacytoid DCs.

In addition, CD34+ cells when cultured with GM-CSF and a variety of cytokines, including IL-4, IL-13, TNF-α, and stem cell factor (SCF), generate DCs with the HLA DR+, CD14- phenotype. These in vitro generated DCs coexpress many accessory molecules and are able to stimulate allogenic T cells.

The culture of CD34+ cord blood cells with GM-CSF and TNF-α generates a subpopulation of cells with some features of DCs and LCs, including expression of CD1a and HLA DR, Birbeck granules, and many costimulatory molecules.

Concluding Remarks

DC phenotypes vary considerably depending on their tissue of localization, their level of maturation, and their degree of activation. It is not known why DCs with different phenotypes are needed in different organs or in different compartments of the same organs. The hallmark of phenotypic differentiation of DCs is the expression of certain surface molecules. As the function of the majority of these surface molecules on DCs are still unknown, it is practically impossible to comment on the actual functional implications of different phenotypes of DCs in vivo.

It is not known whether the phenotype of DCs is decided at the time of their origin or whether they acquire their phenotypic markers after becoming localized in the tissues. For example, it is important to understand whether the so-called putative myeloid DCs of the spleen expressing DEC-205 and CD8α originated as such in the bone marrow or whether different populations of DCs develop these markers after localization in the PALS of the spleen. The impact of the tissue microenvironment on phenotypic diversity of DCs requires further study.

From a functional viewpoint, DCs, or their precursors in human peripheral blood, can be divided into two major phenotypes by their expression of CD11c and CD123, but the functional roles of these antigens are not clear. CD11c-, CD123+ DCs are plasmacytoid DCs or type-1 IFN-producing DCs. It is not clear why the absence of CD11c or the presence of CD123 endows these DCs with a potent type-1 IFN-producing capacity. Similarly, it is not known why these DCs are able to induce polarization to both T helper (Th) 1- and Th2-type immune responses.

However, in some organs, the implications of DC phenotypic diversity are partially understood. DEC-205+ DCs in the spleen may be important for antigen uptake, because DEC-205 is a type of mannose receptor, whereas DEC-205- DCs may have other functions.

From the present state of DC biology, it is apparent that the diverse DC phenotypes have been associated with DC function in a very insignificant way, because function-specific DC markers remain unknown. The future challenge of DC biology lies in finding a relationship between the phenotypic heterogeneity of DCs and their functional diversity. Also, understanding the role of the tissue microenvironment in the phenotypic diversity of DCs is a challenging area of DC research.

Origin and Developmental Aspects of Dendritic Cells

DCs constitute a system of hematopoietic cells that are rare but ubiquitously distributed in different tissues. DCs, their progenitors, or their precursors can be detected in various organs and tissues, for example LCs in the epidermis, DDCs in the dermis, interstitial DCs in various nonlymphoid organs, thymic DCs in the thymus, and circulatory DCs in the blood. A wide range of heterogeneity is evident regarding phenotype, level of maturation, degree of activation, and function. Whether this heterogeneity is determined at the time of origin or is fixed later under the influence of the tissue microenvironment is an open question.

Murine DCs

Development of DCs from Lineage-Negative "Low-CD4 Precursors" in the Murine Thymus

In the murine thymus, an early putative lymphoid-restricted precursor population is called "low-CD4 precursors." This precursor population is negative for markers of hematopoietic lineage, but expresses low levels of CD4 and Thy 1 and very high levels of the hematopoietic progenitor cell marker c-kit. The precursors are able to produce DCs as well as T cells, B cells, and NK cells, and they can differentiate along myeloid and erythroid pathways. However, although they express CD4, they are not committed to the T-cell lineage.

Development of DCs from Progenitors in the Murine Bone Marrow

In murine bone marrow, clonogenic common myeloid progenitors (CMPs) and common lymphoid progenitors (CLPs) have been identified based on their expression of IL-7Rα. The CLPs are lin$^-$, IL-7Rα$^+$, cKit^{low}, and Sca^{low}. These cells can produce all lymphoid cells and some DCs, but no myeloid or erythroid cells.

The CMPs are lin$^-$, IL-7Rα$^-$, cKit$^+$, Sca$^-$, CD34$^+$, and FCRγ^{low}. CMPs can give rise to precursors for megakaryocytes/erythrocytes and for granulocytes/macrophages. CMPs can also produce DCs.

Development of DCs from MHC Class II-Negative Progenitors in Murine Peripheral Blood

DCs can be generated from MHC class II-negative progenitors in murine peripheral blood by culture with GM-CSF. However, if macrophage CSF (M-CSF) or granulocyte CSF (G-CSF) is used, despite the presence of GM-CSF, DCs do not develop, indicating the presence of committed precursors of DCs in the peripheral blood.

Development of LCs from CD34$^+$ Hematopoietic Progenitor Cells

In mice, LCs can be produced from CD34$^+$ HPCs in vitro by culturing with GM-CSF and TNF-α. If transforming growth factor (TGF)-β in added to these cultures, it is possible to get a committed colony of LCs. Among CD34$^+$ progenitor cells, the expression of low levels of IL-3Rα chains or the expression of CLAs defines progenitor cells that can preferentially give rise to LCs in culture. TGF-β plays a critical role in the development of LCs because TGF-β knockout mice lack LCs, but not their precursors. LCs can also be generated from lymphoid-committed CD4^{low} precursors.

Developmental Pathway of CD8α⁻ Myeloid DCs and CD8α⁺ Lymphoid DCs

Although DCs can be generated in vitro from progenitors such as CMP and CLP or from progenitors in the blood, bone marrow, or thymus, recent studies on the developmental pathway of the so-called putative myeloid DCs and putative lymphoid DCs have provided important information regarding the origin of DCs.

First, both $CD8\alpha^+$ lymphoid DCs and $CD8\alpha^-$ myeloid DCs can be generated in vivo after the transfer of $CD4^{low}$ precursors. These data indicate that both myeloid DCs and lymphoid DCs are derived from a common progenitor, which does not support the concept of independent $CD8\alpha^+$ lymphoid-derived and $CD8\alpha^-$ myeloid-derived DC lineages.

Furthermore, it has been shown that more than 70% of $CD8\alpha^-$ myeloid DCs are $CD4^+$. These data suggest that myeloid DCs can be generated from a myeloid precursor within a $CD4^{low}$ precursor population. Alternatively, $CD8\alpha^+$ and $CD8\alpha^-$ DCs may be produced from non-myeloid, nonlymphoid precursors.

It has also been shown that both $CD8\alpha^+$ lymphoid DCs and $CD8\alpha^-$ myeloid DCs can originate from both CMPs and CLPs in both thymus and spleen.

Human DCs

Human DCs originate from $CD34^+$ HPCs. These cells are originally produced in the bone marrow, but they have also been traced to cord blood, peripheral blood, and fetal liver. The human equivalent of mouse CMPs has not been discovered. However, human progenitor cells with features similar to those of murine CLPs have been identified, although the generation of myeloid or lymphoid DCs in human from these progenitor populations is not clear. $CD34^+$ stem cells comprise $CD34^+$ myeloid cells, which also express CD33, and $CD34^+$ lymphoid cells, which express CD10.

Differentiation of DCs from $CD34^+$ Progenitors

$CD34^+$ HPCs obtained from cord blood or bone marrow differentiate into DCs when cultured with GM-CSF and TNF-α. In these cultures, two independent, immature DC intermediates are produced. These intermediates are differentiated by their expression of CD14 and CD1a. $CD14^+$ and $CD1a^-$ intermediates produce DCs when cultured with GM-CSF and TNF-α. The resulting DCs are E-Cadherin⁻ with a comparatively mature phenotype and resemble dermal or lymphoid-organ DCs. Macrophages are generated when these intermediates are cultured with M-CSF, indicating that the $CD14^+$ $CD1a^-$ pathway originated from a myeloid progenitor.

On the other hand, $CD14^-$, $CD1a^+$ intermediates give rise to E-cadherin⁺, langerin⁺ LC-like DCs by a TGF-β-independent pathway. LCs can also be produced by culturing $CD14^+$, $CD1a^-$, $CD11b^-$ fractions with TGF-β.

Another subpopulation of $CD34^+$ HSCs in the peripheral blood is lin⁻, $CD11c^+$. These precursor populations are committed to DC development because they can spontaneously develop into DCs when cultured without added cytokines. $CD34^+$, $CD10^+$ lymphoid-committed stem cells may produce lymphoid DCs when cultured with IL-3.

DCs produced by culturing stem cells are immature, but all of them may be induced to undergo maturation by the presence of various stimulators. TNF-α, dsDNA, lipopolysaccharide (LPS), IFN-γ, and CD40 ligation are the most-used maturation stimuli for these DCs.

Treatment of CD34$^+$ stem cells with G-CSF greatly enhances the yield of DCs. DCs can also be generated by culturing CD34$^+$ stem cells with GM-CSF and TNF-α. But culturing them first with a cytokine cocktail containing IL-3, IL-6, and SCF, and subsequently with GM-CSF and IL-4 results in a tremendous increase in DC numbers.

CD34$^+$ cells in the peripheral blood can be divided into CD34$^+$, CLA$^+$ and CD34$^+$, CLA$^-$ phenotypes. The latter develop into LCs upon culture with GM-CSF and TNF-α.

When human fetal liver is mechanically disrupted, CD34$^+$, lin$^-$, CD38$^{-/dim}$ cells can be collected. A tissue culture system developed by culturing these stem cells in a murine thymic microenvironment yields HLA DR$^+$ DCs, but the yield is too low for practical use. DCs can also be produced by culturing thymic CD34$^+$ CD38$^{-/dim}$ and lin$^-$ cells with GM-CSF, TNF-α, and SCF.

Development of DCs from Precursors in the Peripheral Blood: Monocytes, the Most Widely Used Precursor of DCs

DCs have been developed from PBMCs or CD14$^+$ monocytes and from a monocyte-rich adherent population of PBMCs in vitro by culturing with GM-CSF and IL-4 for variable lengths of time. These DCs have the characteristics of myeloid DCs. Initially, they are immature with respect to both phenotype and function, but they mature when cultured with various combinations of cytokines.

Development of DCs from Precursor Populations Defined by CD11c or ILT3/ILT1

Two distinct populations of DC precursors can be distinguished by their expression of CD11c and CD123 in PBMCs. Myeloid DC precursors (Lin$^-$, HLA DR$^+$ and CD11c$^+$, CD123$^-$) and lymphoid DC precursors (lin$^-$, HLA DR$^+$, CD11c$^-$, CD123$^+$) are separated by using cell sorting techniques. The CD11c$^+$ cells are CD45RO$^+$, express GM-CSF receptor, and have other features of DCs, including expression of CD80 and CD86. These cells convert into myeloid DCs under the influence of GM-CSF and IL-4. Some CD11c$^+$ DCs also express CD1a, and these cells differentiate into LCs in the presence of GM-CSF and TGF-β.

CD11c$^-$ cells express high levels of CD123 (IL-3R) and very low levels of GM-CSF receptor, and they differentiate into plasmacytoid DCs in response to IL-3 and CD40L. IL-4 alone or in combination with IL-10 kills CD11c$^-$ DCs, but that fate can be averted by pretreatment with CD40 L, IFN-γ, or IL-3.

In addition, DC precursors have been classified by their expression of ILT. Lin$^-$, ILT3$^+$, ILT1$^+$ cells appear to mature into CD11c$^+$ DCs, whereas Lin$^-$, ILT3$^+$, ILT1$^-$ cells become CD11c$^-$ DCs.

Differentiation Pathway of Plasmacytoid DCs

The IFN-α developmental pathway produces pre-dendritic cells 2 (Pre-DC2) from human CD34$^+$ HPCs. These cells can be obtained from fetal liver, bone marrow, cord blood, and adult blood. At least four developmental stages have been identified by flow cytometry. The early progenitor cells of Pre-DC2 are lineage⁻, $CD34^+$, $CD45RA^-$, $CD4^+$, $CD123^+$. These cells have high proliferative capacity. Although they are the early progenitors of IFN-producing DCs, they cannot produce type-1 IFN in vitro. The late progenitors of Pre-DC2 express low levels of CD45RA; otherwise they are phenotypically similar to early progenitors of Pre-DC2. This population has very little capacity to produce type-1 IFN in vitro. Pre-DC2 are still positive for CD34 antigen and express higher levels of CD45RA and CD123 compared to early and late progenitors of Pre-DC2. Eventually, Pre-DC2 become negative for CD34 and capable of producing very high levels of type-1 IFN in vitro. However, these cells are almost devoid of proliferative capacity. The culture of pre-DC2 with IL-3R or CD40L produces plasmacytoid DCs.

DCs and Their Lineage Origin

Myeloid and Lymphoid DC Differentiation Pathways and Their Relevance In Vivo

Several studies in vitro have shown that myeloid or lymphoid DCs can be generated from myeloid or lymphoid precursors or from uncommitted precursors. However, the relevance of these findings in vivo is controversial.

For example, both $CD8\alpha^+$ lymphoid DCs and $CD8\alpha^-$ myeloid DCs can be derived in vitro from both myeloid and lymphoid progenitors. LCs can also be generated in vitro from both myeloid and lymphoid precursors. In humans, DCs that express myeloid markers can also be generated from lymphoid precursors.

However, the differentiation of DCs in vivo into myeloid or lymphoid populations under physiological conditions has not been confirmed by in vitro studies. Thus, the derivation of DC subsets in vivo remains an unresolved question.

Scientific Validity of Myeloid and Lymphoid DCs Based on the Expression of CD8α

The initial observation that $CD8\alpha^+$ DCs but not $CD8\alpha^-$ DCs were generated from $CD4^{low}$ lymphoid precursors led to the hypothesis that mouse $CD8\alpha^+$ DCs are lymphoid and $CD8\alpha^-$ DCs are myeloid. However, a recent study showed that both $CD8\alpha^+$ DCs and $CD8\alpha^-$ DCs can be generated from $CD4^{low}$ precursor cells. Later, it was further confirmed that $CD8\alpha^+$ and $CD8\alpha^-$ DCs could both be generated from lymphoid- and myeloid-committed progenitors. Therefore, experimental evidence no longer supports the interpretation that $CD8\alpha^+$ DC and $CD8\alpha^-$ DC are lymphoid and myeloid DCs, respectively, or that they represent different DC lineages.

Dilemma About the Origin of DCs

DCs are derived from bone marrow and they originate from $CD34^+$ HPCs. In vitro culture of $CD34^+$ HPCs leads to the production of almost all types of DCs. The important problem is the characterization of the intermediate precursors. These intermediate precursors may play a dominant role in the production of different subsets of DCs. In fact, the development of DCs has mainly been evaluated in cultures, and very little information is available regarding the implications of these findings in vivo.

DCs display several similarities with monocytes and macrophages with respect to (1) distribution in the lymphoid tissues; (2) morphology; (3) phenotype; (4) enzymatic activities; (5) endocytic and phagocytic activities; and (6) function. These similarities suggested that DCs are of myeloid origin. However, a series of experiments both in vivo and in vitro clearly indicate that DCs can be generated from lymphoid-committed precursors. Therefore, the derivation of different subsets of DCs from myeloid and lymphoid precursors is controversial.

Evidence for a myeloid DC lineage derives, in part, from human and mouse in vitro DC differentiation assays. DCs can be generated from monocytes or intermediate myeloid precursors that retain the capacity to generate macrophages. Bipotential macrophages–DC precursors have been located in mouse bone marrow and in dermal CD11b$^+$ phenotypic cells. Especially, these dermal DC precursors can become DCs after migration to the lymph nodes. These studies gave rise to the concept of myeloid-related DCs.

The first evidence for generation of DCs from lymphoid-committed precursors came from a study of the development of thymic DCs. The earliest murine thymic precursors, namely CD4^{low} precursors, differentiated into T, B, and NK cells as well as CD8α^+ DCs, but not into any sort of myeloid cells. This provided a proof of the origin of lymphoid-related DCs.

The recent discovery of plasmacytoid DCs also supports the concept of lymphoid-related DCs. Plasmacytoid DCs have a strong capacity to produce type-1 IFN, and they mature in the presence of IL-3 and CD40L, becoming functional DCs. These DCs are thought to be lymphoid related because (1) they depend on IL-3, but not on GM-CSF, for survival and differentiation; (2) they express pTα, which upon assembly with T-cell receptor (TCR) β chains form a pre-TCR; and (3) they inhibit development of T and B cells and plasmacytoid DCs from liver precursors transfected with inhibitor of DNA binding (Id) 2 and Id3.

However, a myeloid origin of plasmacytoid DCs should also be considered because CD34$^+$, M-CSF receptor$^+$ progenitors may give rise to plasmacytoid DCs. In mouse, plasmacytoid DCs can be developed from CD11c^{low}, CD11b$^-$, CD8α^- cells of the mouse spleen. Moreover, so-called murine plasmacytoid DCs are CD11c$^+$.

Phenotypic Diversity and the Origin of DCs

CD8α^+ DCs are present in the PALS of the murine spleen and lymph nodes, whereas CD8α^- DCs are located in the marginal zone of the spleen and in the subcapsular sinus of the lymph nodes. It is presumed that DCs in secondary lymphoid organs such as spleen and lymph nodes migrate mainly from nonlymphoid tissues. However, some DCs may migrate directly from the bone marrow and settle in the lymphoid tissues. It is still uncertain whether DCs from all nonlymphoid tissues express CD8α antigen. The natural question arises as to how DCs in the lymphoid tissues acquire CD8α antigens and become localized in a particular compartment of lymphoid tissues. Similarly, questions arise concerning DEC-205$^+$ DCs. LCs do not express CD8α, but CD8α^+ DCs can be traced in local lymph nodes or in the spleen. Although this suggests that the phenotypes of DCs might not be determined at the time of origin, it is difficult to decide whether this inference arises from a poor understanding of putative markers of DC progenitors and DC precursors.

Diversity Regarding Activation and Maturation of DCs and Their Origin

Bone marrow-derived DCs and the precursors or progenitors of DCs are inherently immature owing to their low expression of costimulatory molecules. The activation or maturation of DCs is initiated following capture of microbes, migration of DCs to lymphoid tissues, or localization in a proinflammatory microenvironment. However, the same conditions or criteria may also downregulate the activation of DCs, leading to the production of tolerogenic DCs. How the formation of these so-called immunogenic and tolerogenic DCs is regulated in vivo is not known. Little is understood regarding the nature of the stimuli or the mode of induction of activation and maturation of DCs in situ. However, it is necessary to understand whether different populations of DCs acquire their typical functional capacity during development.

Diversity Regarding Function and Origin of DCs

The most magnificent feature of DCs is their extreme diversity of function. Immature DCs in the nonlymphoid tissues can capture antigens or microbes and become migratory after processing these in their endosomal compartments. They either present antigens for the induction of immunity or simply induce immune tolerance after antigen uptake. They can produce and induce a variety of cytokines that are known to be proinflammatory. Similarly, they can produce cytokines and mediators that are known to be inhibitory in the context of the immune response. Absolutely different from these scenarios, some DCs can also produce type-1 IFN, which is a bridge between innate and adaptive immunity. Most strikingly, the same types of DCs can have completely different functions in vitro, depending on the nature of the stimuli. Thus, it is natural to ask if DC function is determined at the time of their origin and how DCs retain so much plasticity in pursuing their diverse functions.

Concluding Remarks

It is clear that DCs are bone marrow-derived and that they originate from $CD34^+$ HPCs. Different combinations of cytokines are required for their production in vitro. However, current information from humans and mice does not support a conclusive definition of the physiological differentiation pathways that generate DCs in vivo. Several factors may account for this. First, several lines of experimental evidence suggest that in vivo differentiation of a particular DC population from a myeloid or a lymphoid progenitor might differ from its generation under experimental conditions. When murine DCs develop in vivo in irradiated mice from their precursor populations, the physiological developmental potential of a defined precursor might be altered by this experimental situation; when a precursor population is isolated by irradiation, the nature of the precursor is altered by handling during isolation. This may induce a nonphysiological differentiation behavior owing to partial reversion of its lineage commitment. Thus, lymphoid-committed precursors may give rise to myeloid DCs and vice versa.

In humans, when DCs are differentiated by using a complex combination of cytokines, conditions are no longer physiological. It is instead a nonphysiological differentiation pathway of defined committed precursors. Obviously, these situations would be further complicated if bipotential differentiation of myeloid and lymphoid precursors is real.

All these factors are highly important in clinical contexts, where DCs are studied to understand pathological processes and used for therapeutic purposes. Several studies are in progress on DC phenotypes and functions under pathological conditions, including in malignancies. In most of these studies, DCs were enriched from several tissues in vitro. The functioning of in vitro generated DCs is either impaired or exacerbated under pathological conditions compared with that of DCs from so-called normal individuals. Based on the results from these studies, DC-based therapy has begun for several pathological conditions, and many such therapies will be implemented in the future. It is now evident that DCs used for functional characterization or for DC-based therapy are not truly representative of DCs in vivo. Investigators obtain terminally differentiated DCs for characterization. However, it is very likely that the impairment of DCs was initiated at specific times during their origin or differentiation. For example, infection and low functioning of pre-DC2 or NIPCs have been reported in cases of HIV infection. Four known developmental stages of NIPCs are now known. However, it is not clear at which stage of differentiation, pre-DC2 were invaded by HIV. Similarly, defective functioning of in vitro generated DCs in malignancies has been reported. However, it is unknown how malignant cells affect the differentiation and functioning of DCs in vivo. Indeed, understanding of these factors is vitally important for the development of therapies and for understanding pathological processes.

Functions of Dendritic Cells

APC Function of DCs

DCs are professional antigen-presenting cells in vivo. In addition to the capture and processing of microbes and their Ags, DCs also perform a variety of other functions. DCs may be committed to some of these functions during their development from progenitor and precursor cells. On the other hand, DCs may acquire some of their activities after capturing antigens. The tissue microenvironment may also influence several DC functions. Although other APCs can perform some of the functions of DCs, DCs are called professional APCs owing to their capacity to induce activation, proliferation, and differentiation of naive T cells.

The diverse nature of DCs with respect to phenotypes, stages of maturation, and degree of activation indicate that DCs are multifunctional. Some immature DCs are designed to induce immunity, whereas others may be tolerogenic. The functions of mature DCs may be different in nonlymphoid and lymphoid tissues. The functions of DCs in nonlymphoid parenchymal tissues differ from those in lymphoid tissues or in the blood or bone marrow. Several subtypes of DCs have been detected both in vivo and in vitro. Although we do not yet understand completely the phenotypic diversity and functions of DCs, many new functions of DCs have been found in vitro. Furthermore, DC progenitors and precursors not only are destined to become DCs, but also exhibit other important functional potentials, especially in vitro. The most important limitation to our understanding is that, even though the bulk of DC functions have been studied in vitro, the real functional potential of DCs still needs to be explored in vivo.

Given all these practical limitations regarding our understanding the functions of DCs, it is nevertheless well understood that as professional APCs, DCs perform certain functions in an orderly fashion for the induction of an immune response. First, DCs recognize and capture microbes or their antigens or apoptotic cells in the tissue of their localization. After the captured cells or molecules are internalized, subsequent steps depend on the nature of the internalized materials. In certain circumstances, DCs cleave the antigens and express antigenic peptides with self-MHC molecules. These DCs then migrate to lymphoid tissues to present the antigenic peptide to clonally selected T lymphocytes. Under certain conditions, DCs, T cells, and B cells may also form an immunogenic synapse. These interactions lead to the formation of activated lymphocytes and the maturation or activation of DCs. The activated lymphocytes perform their assigned effector functions in the context of cellular or humoral immunity.

However, this scenario may be completely different if DCs in the tissue determine, after internalization of an apoptotic cell or microbial agent or certain Ags, that the induction of an immune response is unnecessary. Moreover, the scenario may be altered if tolerogenic DCs engulf microbes or their antigens. The following sections describe the typical APC functioning of DCs (Fig. 2.3).

Antigen Recognition Functions of DCs

The single most important event that determines the subsequent cascade of antigen presentation is the recognition of antigens or antigen-bearing microbes by DCs. It is now evident that the immune system recognizes danger signals from the host. In this regard, the most relevant receptors are pattern-recognition receptors. These receptors can bind a range of molecules with structural patterns common to the surfaces of many microbes but absent from the surfaces of mammalian cells. Macrophage mannose receptor and other lectin-like molecules on DCs may bind with molecules on the surfaces of microbes.

Another family of pattern-recognition receptors includes the Toll-like receptors (TLRs). TLRs, which are phylogenetically well conserved, are type 1 transmembrane receptors and major pattern-recognition receptors for various pathogen-associated molecular patterns in the innate immune system. To date, ten TLRs have been described in the literature. Human monocyte-derived DCs and CD11c$^+$ blood myeloid DCs express TLR1, TLR2, TLR4, TLR5, TLR6, and TLR8. On the other hand, CD11c$^-$, CD123$^+$ plasmacytoid DCs express TLR7 and TLR9 and low TLR1, TLR6, and TLR10.

Very little is known regarding the expression of recognition molecules on other DC populations, especially their expression on DCs in nonlymphoid tissues. Similarly, there is a paucity of information regarding the expression of recognition molecules on different subsets of DCs. It is not known whether immunogenic or tolerogenic DCs exhibit similar types of recognition molecules. Some TLR ligands are known, but their interactions with DCs in vivo remain to be elucidated.

In addition to the recognition of Ags by pathogen recognition receptors on DCs, altered tissue microenvironments may also play a role in Ag recognition by DCs.

Antigen recognition
1) Pattern-recognition molecules
2) Toll-like receptors

Antigen capture and internalization
1) Macropinocytosis
2) FC-receptor-mediated
3) Mannose and C-type lectin receptor-mediated
4) Engulfing of apoptotic bodies

Loading and formation of MHC–Ag complex
1) Complex formation with MHC class II antigen
2) Complex formation with MHC class I antigen

Activation and maturing DCs
1) Pathogen-related molecules; LPS, bacterial DNA, dsRNA
2) Mucosal milieu and cytokines such as TNF-α, IL-6, IL-10, TGF-β, prostaglandins
3) Loss of endocytic and phagocytic apparatus
4) Upregulation of costimulatory molecules such as CD86, CD80, CD40, CD58
5) Shift in lysosomal compartment; Downregulation of CD68 and upregulation of DC-LAMP
6) Alteration in MIIC

Migration of DC
1) Downregulation of CCR6 and upregulation of CCR7

Ag presentation/T-cell activation/survival and functioning of activated lymphocytes
1) Immunogenic synapse at the lymphoid tissue
2) Mature DCs by producing and inducing cytokines and mediators

Fig. 2.3. The cellular and molecular basis of DC function. DCs act as sentinels of the immune system and recognize antigens or other entities by their receptors. DCs are also able to recognize alterations to the microenvironment in which they reside. After capturing and internalizing antigens or other agents, these agents may be routed to the antigen-processing pathway or they may localize in DCs. The peptide MHC complex is expressed by DCs, and then these maturing DCs migrate to the lymphoid tissues, where they present antigenic peptides to lymphocytes. DCs also undergo maturation in the lymphoid tissues, and mature DCs are readily detectable there. *MHC*, major histocompatibility complex; *LPS*, lipopolysaccavide; *TNF*, tumor necrosis factor; *DC-LAMP*, dendritic cell lysosome-associated membrane protein; *MIIC*, major histocompatibility complex class II-rich compartment; *CCR*, CC chemokine receptor

Most importantly, it is not known whether the impaired recognition of Ags by DCs underlies defects in the immune response. It will be interesting to study how apoptotic and cancer cells are recognized by DCs.

Antigen Capture Function of DCs

After the recognition of microbes or their antigens, the next important function of DCs is their capture and internalization. Immature DCs can efficiently internalize a diverse array of antigens for processing and loading onto class II MHC molecules because of their high endocytic activities. Antigen capture by immature DCs is mediated by four distinct mechanisms.
Macropinocytosis. Macropinocytosis is a cytoskeleton-dependent fluid-phase type of endocytosis mediated by membrane ruffling and the formation of large vesicles

(1–3 μm). In DCs, macropinocytosis is constitutive, and enables a single cell to take up a large volume of fluid (half of a cell volume per hour).

Fcγ and Fcε Receptor-Mediated Antigen Capture. Initially, it was thought that DCs lacked Fc receptors; however, several types of Fc receptors have now been detected on various populations of DCs. Fc receptors allow the specific uptake of opsonized antigen. Fresh blood DCs express both CD32 (FcγRII) and CD64 (FcγRI) but not CD16 (FcγRIII). Similarly, human LCs express CD32 and CD64.

Human epidermal DCs, but not other DCs, express FcεR1. The FcεR1 on human epidermis contains α and γ chains but lacks β chains. This receptor probably allows LCs to maximize antigen uptake via a specific IgE.

Antigen Capture by Mannose Receptor and DEC-205. DCs express a type of mannose receptor that contains multiple carbohydrate-binding domains and is involved in the internalization of a type of glycoprotein. One of the major differences between Fc receptors and mannose receptors lies in the fact that Fc receptors are usually degraded with their cargo; however, a mannose receptor releases its ligand at endosomal pH and is recycled. This gives mannose receptors supremacy in uptake and small numbers of receptors accumulate many ligands.

Another endocytic receptor is DEC-205, an integral membrane protein homologous to the mannose receptor. DEC-205 and its antigenic ligands are rapidly taken up by means of coated pits and vesicles. Then, they are delivered to a multivesicular endosomal compartment. This endosomal compartment resembles class II MHC-containing vesicles. DEC-205 is expressed on most mouse DCs, including LCs, but its expression is high on so-called less-activated lymphoid DCs. As the expression of DEC-205 on tissue DCs is very limited, the precise role of these DCs in the uptake of Ags in vivo remains to be elucidated. However, as the expression of DEC-205 can be upregulated according to the status of inflammation of the peripheral tissues, DEC-205 may play an important role in the capture of Ags when the Ags are presented along with inflammatory stimuli.

Engulfment of Apoptotic Bodies by DCs. One of the major functions of DCs under steady-state or physiological conditions is to induce immune tolerance. Cross priming by DCs requires the uptake of apoptotic bodies. Thus, internalization of apoptotic bodies by DCs appears to be a highly efficient machinery for maintaining homeostasis. DCs preferentially use the vitronectin receptor and the CD36/thrombospondin receptor for engulfing apoptotic bodies. Engulfment of apoptotic bodies causes the concentration of intracellular free Ca^{2+} to increase.

The engulfment of Ags from necrotic bodies depends on the nature of the necrotic tissues. If the Ags are free, they are considered nominal Ags. However, if they are opsonized, an Fc receptor might play a role in antigen capture.

Function of DCs Regarding the Formation of MHC Complexes

MHC Class II Loading. Following internalization of antigens, microbes, or apoptotic bodies, DCs must present these antigens to T cells. To do so, DCs first fulfill the other requirements for antigen presentation by synthesizing and expressing high levels of class II MHC antigens. The intracellular class II MHC is found in both late endocytic compartments and in early endosomal compartments in DCs. In DCs, the majority of the intracellular class II MHC is found in late endocytic structures with numerous internal membrane vesicles and sheets. The major MHC class II-rich compartment (MIIC) contains newly synthesized MHC class II molecules that are targeted to this structure by their invariant chains. It also contains HLA DM molecules. A major change in the MIIC occurs during DC maturation. In early DCs, class II MHC molecules are localized to lysosomal compartments; in intermediate DCs, class II MHC molecules are accumulated in distinctive nonlysosomal vesicles; and in mature DCs, MHC–peptide complexes are present on the surfaces of DCs for long periods. This allows prolonged interaction between DCs and rare antigen-specific T lymphocytes.

MHC Class I Loading. MHC class I loading is critical for the activation of $CD8^+$ T cells. DCs can capture exogenous antigens for presentation to MHC class I molecules. This ensures an efficient generation of cytotoxic T lymphocytes (CTLs), even against viral and tumor antigens, which are expressed only on nonprofessional APCs. For class I loading, two pathways are required: (1) unconventional post-Golgi loading of MHC class I and (2) involvement of a classical transporter-associated antigen processing (TAP) loading mechanism. Thus, a functional TAP pathway is required for efficient loading of the class I MHC. The peptides for the class I MHC on DCs are derived from nonreplicating microbes, soluble proteins, and apoptotic cells.

Activation and Maturation Functions of DCs

After microbes or their antigens are internalized by DCs and programmed to MHC class II or class I molecules, an antigen—MHC complex is ultimately expressed on the surfaces of the DCs. Several molecules, including CD40, TNF-R, and IL 1R, have been shown to activate DCs and to trigger their transition from immature antigen-capturing DCs to maturing antigen-presenting DCs. DC maturation is a continuous process initiated in the periphery upon antigen encounter or by inflammatory cytokines and completed during DC—T cell interaction. Numerous factors induce or regulate DC maturation, including (1) pathogen-related molecules such as LPS, bacterial DNA, and double-stranded RNA; (2) the balance between proinflammatory and anti-inflammatory signals in the local microenvironment, including TNF-α, IL-1, IL-6, IL-10, TGF-β, and prostaglandins; and (3) T-cell-derived signals. The maturation process is associated with several coordinated events: (1) loss of endocytic and phagocyte receptors; (2) upregulation of costimulatory molecules CD40, CD58, CD80, and CD86; (3) changes in morphology; (4) a shift in lysosomal compartments with downregulation of CD68 and upregulation of DC lysosome-associated membrane protein (DC-LAMP); and (5) changes in MHC class II compartments.

Morphological changes accompanying DC maturation include a loss of adhesive structure, cytoskeleton reorganization, and the acquisition of greater cellular motility. The actin-binding protein fascin p55 may play a role in controlling DC maturation. Immune regulatory tyrosine-based inhibitory motif characteristics of immunoglobulin superfamily members and membrane lectins may regulate DC maturation and activation.

Migration of DCs

Several studies have shown that DCs leave the nonlymphoid organs through the afferent lymph. Pathogen products LPS, IL-1, and TNF-α, all mediators of DC maturation, also favor the migration of DC. Several chemokines are also involved in coordinated migration of DCs to lymphoid tissue. After antigen uptake, inflammatory stimuli turn off the response of immature DCs to macrophage inflammatory protein (MIP)-3α through either receptor downregulation or receptor desensitization, depending on autocrine chemokine production. Maturing DCs escape from the local gradient of MIP-3α. Upon maturation, DCs upregulate a single known chemokine receptor, CCR7, and acquire responsiveness to MIP-3β. Accordingly, maturing DCs leave the inflamed tissue and enter the lymph stream apparently directed by secondary lymphoid-tissue chemokines (SLCs). Mature DCs entering the draining lymph node will be driven into the paracortical area in response to the production of MIP-3β and SLCs, allowing the amplification or persistence of a chemotactic signal. Mature DCs may become a source of MIP-3β and SLCs, thus also allowing amplification or persistence of a chemotactic signal. Because two chemokines can attract mature DCs and naive T cells, they are likely to play a key role in helping Ag-bearing DCs to encounter specific T cells. This has been proved in an SLC-mutant mouse and in CCR7-deficient mice, both of which had a specific deficiency respecting T-cell and DC homing into the lymph nodes. Upon encountering T cells, which takes place not only in the secondary lymphoid organs but also at the site of tissue injury, DCs receive additional signals from CD40L, which induces the release of chemokines such as IL-8 and fractalkine, and macrophage-derived chemokines that attract lymphocytes.

LCs in both humans and mice migrate in response to IL-1β and TNF-α. IL-1β is also produced by LCs, and thus regulates the migration of LCs in an autocrine fashion because LCs also express IL-1βR. IL-1β also acts in paracrine fashion by producing TNF-α. Mobilization of LCs by these cytokines might be inhibited by IL-4. TGF-β, which is required for LC development in vivo and in vitro, prevents maturation of LCs in response to IL-1, TNF-α, and LPS but not to CD40 ligation.

The molecular mechanism of LC migration is becoming clear. During migration, LCs downregulate E-cadherin, which favors detachment from keratinocytes and adherence to basement membrane. They also secret type IV collagenase for crossing basement membrane. LCs migrate from the epidermis into dermal lymphatic vessels and out of the tissue, and the migration is accompanied by phenotypic and functional maturation of the cells. Similarly, migration of DCs from the gut to regional lymph nodes has been shown.

Antigen Presentation and T-Cell Activation

Experimental evidence shows that DCs present antigens to T cells. Soluble antigen-pulsed DCs elicit potent Ag-specific immune responses, and DC-T helper cell inter-actions in the PALS have been demonstrated by immunohistochemistry. In the presence of soluble Ags, T helper cells primed by DCs can interact with B cells and may stimulate Ag-specific B lymphocytes to produce antibodies. DCs are equally important in priming naive T cells. In vitro, DCs can stimulate proliferation of allo-genic T cells directly in the absence of T cell help. They can also generate Ag-specific CTLs from naive T cells. Strong CTL responses can be induced in vivo by injection of mice with Ag-bearing DCs, including allogenic DCs, peptide-pulsed DCs, protein-loaded DCs, DCs transfected with DNA, DCs expressing virally encoded antigens, and DCs pulsed with RNA. Although DCs can induce CTLs, they also require T cell help.

According to the traditional model of CTL activation, CD4 and CD8 cells recognize Ags on the same DCs. However, conditioned DCs become a temporal bridge between T helper cells and T killer cells. DCs are conditioned by interacting with T helper cells. These DCs have information from Th cells and polarize the CTLs to become killer cells. Mature DCs appear to be essential to ensure the survival of naive CD4 T cells and immune T cell memory.

Cellular Mechanisms of Diversity of DC Function

Distinct T Helper Subsets Induce Distinct T Helper Responses

In human, CD11c$^+$ DCs polarize naive T cells toward a Th1 pathway, whereas CD11c$^-$ DCs induce T cells to predominantly produce Th2 cytokines. The polarization by CD11c$^-$ DCs is dependent on their maturational status. Recently, it has been shown that CD11$^-$ DCs can also polarize T cells toward Th1, depending on the nature of the stimulating agent. CD11C$^+$ DCs induce IL-12 from T cells.

In mice, splenic CD8$^+$ DCs prime naive T cells to produce IL-12. CD8$^-$ myeloid DCs induce Th2 cytokines from naive T cells. GM-CSF, which preferentially mobilizes myeloid DCs, induces IgG1 secretion, whereas Flt-3L, which induces both myeloid and lymphoid DCs, induces IgG2a antibodies, a Th1 signature.

The mechanism by which myeloid DCs induce Th2 cytokines is not known, although IL-13 and IL-6 are good candidate molecules. The involvement of CD80 and CD86 in Th1 and Th2 polarization is not clear, but in general CD80 promotes Th1 and CD86 induces Th2 polarization.

Plasticity of DC Function

DCs exhibit considerable plasticity in their ability to skew Th responses. DCs that normally induce Th1 profiles can be converted to Th2-skewing cells when treated with IL-10 and TGF-β, or with steroids or prostaglandin E2. DCs isolated from different organs also induce different Th responses. Rat DCs from PP elicit Th2 responses, whereas those from spleen induce Th1 responses. The mechanism underlying these functional differences is currently unknown. These observations suggest that distinct immunological outcomes would result from oral versus systemic administration of Ags. Thus, adjuvants such as LPS and Flt 3L enhance immunological tolerance to orally administered antigens, but abrogate tolerance to systemic antigens.

DC plasticity is also reflected in their differentiation, that is, processing, presentation, and degradation, which may determine the fate of Ags. This is exemplified by the ability of macrophages to differentiate to DCs, a pathway that may permit high antigen capture (macrophage) and presentation (DC). The final signal for DC maturation and differentiation may be provided during the migration of DCs across the endothelial barrier between the inflamed tissues and the lymphatics.

Dendritic Cells and Tolerance

In mice, thymic DCs are capable of mediating the negative selection of T cells in fetal organ culture and against superantigens in vivo. In addition, thymic DCs can induce tolerance to myelin basic protein and can limit the development of experimental autoimmune encephalitis.

The role of DCs in establishing peripheral tolerance has not been formally demonstrated. In fact, available evidence suggests that DCs can abrogate T-cell tolerance against soluble antigens, viral antigens, tumors, and transplant antigens in neonates. However, it has been shown that lymphoid DCs can limit the proliferation of T cells. The lymphoid DCs appear to kill a proportion of the activated T cells and to limit cytokine production by CD8$^+$ T cells. DCs are important in inducing transplant tolerance through the development of microchimerism.

DCs as Effectors of Innate Immunity

DCs at different stages of differentiation can regulate effectors of innate immunity such as NK cells and natural killer T (NKT) cells. Both direct cell—cell interactions and indirect cytokine-mediated interactions have been implicated. Precursors of CD11c$^-$ DCs can activate NK cells by releasing IFN-α, thereby inducing increased antiviral and antitumor immunity. DCs at a later stage of differentiation may regulate the activity of NK cells and NKT cells through the release of cytokines such as IL-12, IL-15, and IL-18.

Both murine and human NKT cells produce high amounts of IFN-γ or IL-4 and may thus determine the type of immune response. On recognition of an α-galactosylceramide/CD1d complex, NKT cells release IFN-γ. However, DC subsets differentially regulate NKT cytokine profiles, with monocyte-derived DCs producing IFN-γ release, whereas plasmacytoid DCs polarize NKT cells to IL-4 production.

DCs can also activate NK cells, directly or indirectly. In murine tumor models, DC transfer or in vivo mobilization with Flt-3L may account for the potent antitumor activity of Flt-3L. DCs can trigger NK cells, through the release of IL-12, to CD28-dependent and -independent cytotoxicity.

Signaling Pathways in DC Differentiation and Maturation

DC progenitors and precursors derived from CD34$^+$ HPCs localize in various tissues, including blood and bone marrow. Immature DCs localized in nonlymphoid tissues undergo maturation in response to the uptake of Ags or inflammatory stimuli. However, specific biochemical pathways and genes whose expression mediates the differentiation of progenitors to DCs and the maturation of those DCs are largely undefined. By using two approaches, DNA microarrays and proteomics, insights have been gained into the signaling pathways during DC differentiation and maturation.

Monocyte-derived DCs are a good model for studying these signaling pathways. Using oligonucleotide arrays, RNA transcript levels for different genes expressed during DC differentiation were determined on day 1 (CD14$^+$ monocytes), after 7 days of GM-CSF/IL-4 treatment (immature DCs), and after 14 days of GM-CSF/IL-4 plus TNF-α treatment (mature DCs). Transcripts for approximately 40% of the 6300 unique genes assessed were detected in all cell populations tested. However, the expression levels of several genes differed during DC differentiation and maturation by 2.5-fold or greater. The regulated genes were mostly involved in cell adhesion, motility, growth control, regulation of the immune response, antigen presentation, transcription, and signal transduction.

During DC differentiation, the transcript levels of the genes for CD14, CD163, and C5a anaphylatoxin receptor (CD88) were strongly downregulated. On the other hand, those of cell surface proteins MHC class II, CD1a, CD1b, CD1c, CD36, CD59, CD83, CD86, and CCR7 were upregulated.

A large number of genes encoding for proteins involved in cell adhesion and motility were regulated during DC differentiation. Expression of genes for galectin-2, CD11a/LFA-1α, ninjurin 1, MacMARCKS, syndecan 2, CD44E, and presenilin 1 was downregulated. Expression of secreted proteins involved in cell motility, autotaxin-t, and semaphorin E, was upregulated. The decrease in the expression of genes for integrins and cell adhesion molecules and the increase in the expression of genes for proteins involved in cell motility might have an effect on the enhanced migration properties of DCs compared with their precursors.

Differentiation of DCs was also accompanied by differential expression of genes involved in the immune response. The expression of genes encoding anti-inflammatory proteins such as cyclophilin C and TSG-6 was upregulated, whereas that of genes encoding proinflammatory cytokines and their receptors, such as prointerleukin-1, TNF-α, CD163, C5a anaphylatoxin receptor, IL-6 receptor, and TNF receptor were downregulated. Moreover, the expression of a set of chemokines belonging to the IL-8 superfamily such as CTAPIII, MIP2-, MIP2-, ENA78, PF4, and IL-8 was downregulated. Osteopontin, a key cytokine involved in T-lymphocyte activation was upregulated. The maturation of DCs was accompanied by the upregulation of Mac-2 binding protein, which stimulates NK-cell activities, and induces the secretion of IL-2. Upregulation of TGF-β was also observed during DC maturation.

Expression of genes for interferon regulatory factor 4 (IRF-4), C/EBPa, mrg1, PPARg, TRIP7, swine leukocyte antigen (SLA), Rap1GAP, cAMP-dependent protein kinase, IP3 protein kinase B, cyclophilin C, and cyclins A1, D2, G2, and H was increased during maturation. Expression of IRF-7A, TAL2, NAP-2, EGF-response factor 2, CtBP, IEX-1, SAP49, HRH1, I-B alpha, Fyb, Net, and cyclophilin F genes was decreased. Of these genes, IRF-4 and IRF-7 are of particular interest. IRF-7 is traditionally involved in the activation of type-1 IFN and differentiation of monocytes into macrophages. The decrease in IRF-7 during DC differentiation versus increased expression in macrophage differentiation indicate a critical role for IRF-7 at the crossroads between macrophage and DC differentiation from monocytes.

There was marked upregulation of CD36 as well as of the lipid-binding proteins fatty acid-binding protein (FABP) 3, FABP4, FABP5, CRABPII, and acyl-CoA-binding protein (ACBP) during differentiation. Upregulation of FABPs occurred simultaneously with strong downregulation of the S100 proteins, myeloid-related protein (MRP) 8 and MRP14.

Proteomics Applied to DC Differentiation and Maturation

To identify protein changes during the differentiation and maturation of monocyte-derived DCs, total proteins were extracted and protein spots were selected whose intensities changed by 2.5-fold or greater during DC differentiation or maturation. One study found a set of 37 related proteins. The proteins identified were members of specific families, including chaperones, Ca^{2+} binding proteins, FABPs, and structural proteins. Expression of three members of the FABP family, FABP4, FABP5, and ACBP, was highly increased after 7 days of culture of monocytes. The increases in protein levels were similar to the previously observed increases in the RNA levels of these genes. In accordance with the upregulation of FABP4 and FABP5, a strong downregulation of two members of the S100 family, MRP14 and MRP8, was seen. MRP14 and MRP8 downregulation was progressive during DC differentiation and maturation, culminating in a 9- and 12-fold decrease, respectively. Again, the results obtained for the RNA and protein levels were highly concordant.

Several proteins known for their chaperone activity, including heat shock protein (hsp) 73, hsp27, and calreticulin, were also regulated during DC differentiation. Hsp70 enhances antigen uptake by immature DC precursors. Upregulation of hsp73 protein, related to the hsp70 family, during DC differentiation was also observed. Hsp73 has been recently reported to bind specifically to the cell surfaces of monocytic and dendritic cells and to be internalized spontaneously by receptor-mediated endocytosis. In addition, murine hsp73 has been recently reported to accumulate in exosomes from immature DCs. Increased hsp27 expression in DCs may therefore play a protective role against cytotoxicity.

In contrast to hsp27 and hsp73, the cognate chaperone protein calreticulin was downregulated during DC differentiation owing to posttranslational modification. Calreticulin was mostly downregulated during DC maturation. Calreticulin participates in the assembly of MHC class I along with other peptides and β 2-microglobulin in the endoplasmic reticulum, a process required for the presentation of antigenic peptides to CTLs at the cell surface. In addition, it has recently been reported that calreticulin elicits tumor- and peptide-specific immunity. Calreticulin displays in vivo peptide-binding activity and can elicit CTL responses against bound peptides. Discrepancies were found between the protein and gene expression data for vimentin, hsp27, and calreticulin.

In summary, DCs acquire their functions during differentiation and maturation through the programmed expression of specific proteins. Both genomics, relying on the quantitative analysis of mRNAs, and proteomics, relying on the quantitative analysis and identification of proteins, are needed to gain valid insights into signal transduction during DC differentiation and maturation. Information on protein expression levels cannot be obtained simply by examining expression at the RNA level. The proteomics approach is also appropriate for identifying posttranslational modifications, which may regulate protein function. For example, during DC differentiation, MHC class II molecules are synthesized but not stably expressed on the cell surface. However, fully mature DCs stably express MHC class II molecules on the cell surface, and biosynthetic and endocytic traffic ceases.

Oligonucleotide array and proteomics analyses have uncovered novel genes and proteins with potential roles in DC function, differentiation, and maturation. Microarray analysis has identified important changes in genes involved in cell adhesion and motility, the immune response, and growth control, as well as lipid metabolism. Following the simultaneous analysis of several thousand genes at the mRNA level, the challenge is to efficiently utilize this information to develop a better understanding of DC function. Genes and proteins found to be selectively expressed in DCs may provide further understanding of the biological function of DCs in host defense systems and of the mechanisms of antigen processing and presentation.

Concluding Remarks

DCs do not represent a homogeneous cell population, and they are highly versatile. Although originally derived from CD34$^+$ HPCs, the final differentiation of DCs can be induced either from bipotential progenitors or from committed progenitors. The tissue microenvironment where DCs are localized might also influence their terminal differentiation and functional capabilities.

In addition to phenotypic diversity, DCs at variable stages of maturation can be detected from most tissues and organs. DCs, in their progenitor and precursor forms, are readily detectable in vivo. Some do not have any DC-like function (monocytes or CD14$^+$ DC precursors), whereas others perform highly specialized functions (Pre-DC2). Some are immature, and others are mature. Some are assigned to the induction of immunity, whereas others are committed to the induction of tolerance.

The functions of DCs are manifold. They can recognize, capture, and internalize microbes, apoptotic cells, or Ags. The uptake of these cells or molecules causes activation of the DCs, which then migrate to lymphoid tissues and activate T cells. All these roles are APC functions of DCs. However, DCs have many effector functions as well. They produce cytokines and induce lymphocytes to produce cytokines and chemokines.

Although several studies on the phenotypes and origin of DCs have been carried out, the most important aspect of DCs in clinical contests is the relationship between the DC function and the initiation and progression of disease. As APCs, DCs perform a series of functions (Fig. 2.3). Most important is whether impaired functions of DCs in any of these areas lead to pathological processes. The impaired functioning of a bulk population of DCs generated in vitro from tissues from a diseased person has already inspired optimism regarding the use of hyperactivated or tolerogenic DCs for therapy. Also, several attempts have been made to stimulate the function of DCs in vivo by several agents. However, a proper DC-based therapy can only be evolved if the functional impairment of DCs in a particular pathological condition is understood. If defective recognition of Ags leads to persistent infection, there should be a way to stimulate the recognition process of DCs. If instead we activate those DCs, there is little hope of achieving beneficial effects. On the other hand, if tumor-specific lymphocytes are unable to survive in a cancer microenvironment owing to a paucity of activated DCs, then supplying mature DCs or inducing DC maturation will be the treatment of choice.

In conclusion, understanding the nature of the defective functioning of DCs in a particular pathological process will make it possible to develop a DC-based therapy for that process. That should be the aim of DC biologists and clinicians in the 21st century.

Recommended Readings

Ardavin C, del Hoyo GM, Martin P et al. (2001) Origin and differentiation of dendritic cells. Trends Immunol 22:691–700

Banchereau J, Steinman RM (1998) Dendritic cells and the control of immunity. Nature 392:245–252

Banchereau J, Briere F, Cauz C et al. (2000) Immunobiology of dendritic cells. Annu Rev Immunol 18:767–818

Bell D, Young JW, Banchereau J (1999) Dendritic cells. Adv Immunol 73:255–323

Blom B, Ligtart SJWC, Schotte R et al. (2002) Development of origin of Pre-DC2. Human Immunol 63:1072–1080

Hart DNJ (1997) Dendritic cells: unique leukocyte populations which control the primary immune response. Blood 90:3245–3287

Lipscomb MF, Matsen BJ (2002) Dendritic cells: immune regulators in health and disease. Physiol Rev 82:97–130

Lodge MT, Thomson AW (2001) Dendritic cells. Academic Press. San Diego, CA, USA, pp 299–422

Manz M, Traver D, Akashi K et al. (2001) Dendritic cell development from common myeloid progenitors. Ann N Y Acad Sci 938:167–173

Manz MG, Traver D, Miyamoto T et al. (2001) Dendritic cell potentials of early lymphoid and myeloid progenitors. Blood 97:3333–3341

Martin P, del Hoyo GM, Anjuere F et al. (2000) Concept of lymphoid versus myeloid dendritic cell lineages revisited: both CD8α⁻ and CD8α⁺ dendritic cells are generated from CD4^{low} lymphoid-committed precursors. Blood 96:2511–2519

O'Keeffe M, Hochrein H, Vremec D et al. (2003) Dendritic cell precursor populations of mouse blood: identification of the murine homologous of human blood plasmacytoid pre-DC2 and CD11c⁺ DC1 precursors. Blood 101:1453–1459

Shortman K (2000) Dendritic cells: multiple subtypes, multiple origins, multiple functions. Immunol Cell Biol 78:161–165

Siegel FP, Kadowaki N, Shodell M et al. (1999) The nature of the principle type-1 interferon-producing cells in human blood. Science 284:1835–1837

Steinman RM (1991) The dendritic cell system and its role in immunogenicity. Annu Rev Immunol 9:271–296

3. Interactions Between Dendritic Cells and Infectious Agents

Dendritic Cells in Innate and Adaptive Immunity

One of the main characteristics of the evolutionary process is the development of highly sophisticated defense mechanisms for the survival of human beings and other living organisms in hostile environments. There are two such defense systems in higher primates: the innate and adaptive immune responses.

The innate immune system is the first line of defense encountered by invading pathogens. It is composed of bone marrow-derived cells such as neutrophils, macrophages, natural killer (NK) cells and non-bone-marrow-derived cells such as epithelial cells and fibroblasts. All of these cells may produce antimicrobial factors. Macrophages and neutrophils can phagocytose, and NK cells can cause microbe-infected cells to lyse. The induction of innate immunity is quick (from a few minutes to a few hours), and the cells of the innate immune system attack pathogens in a simple way.

In contrast, the adaptive immune system has evolved to provide a more adaptive and highly specific defense response to pathogenic agents, antigens, tumor cells, and possibly to all entities which are nonself and dangerous to the host. The adaptive immune system also possesses the unique ability to induce tolerance to self-structures and possibly to nondangerous stimuli. It takes from several days to several months to develop the effector limb of adaptive immunity. Different types of cells usually participate in the afferent and efferent immune responses of the adaptive immune system.

For a long time, immunologists have known of the existence of innate and adaptive immunity, although only recently have the cellular and molecular mechanisms of these immune responses started to become clear. In this chapter, I provide a comprehensive overview of the roles of antigen-presenting dendritic cells (DCs) during the induction of innate and adaptive immune responses to infectious agents.

In the early 1970s, when Steinman and Cohn first discovered DCs, these cells were shown to be primarily responsible for the induction of adaptive immune responses. Although macrophages and B cells were regarded as functional antigen-presenting cells (APCs), they have other committed functions and do not fulfill the essential criteria of professional APCs. Professional APCs should be able to recognize Ags, microbes, tumor cells, and other nonself and harmful agents. They must have the capacity to capture and internalize these agents. Professional APCs should also be able to process the internalized materials. Antigenic peptides should be routed to the surface of the DCs along with self-major histocompatibility complex (MHC) antigens.

At this stage, DCs become migratory and move to lymphoid organs to interact with lymphocytes. After the discovery and functional characterization of DCs, it became apparent that DCs are the initiators, propagators, and regulators of the adaptive immune response by virtue of their capacity to recognize, capture, process, and present antigens, tumor cells, and apoptotic cells in vivo.

Only recently have the different functions of DCs in innate immunity become apparent, although several investigators have long predicted a role for DCs in the innate immune response. From the ontogenetic point of view, DCs share a common developmental pathway with cells of the monocyte and macrophage lineages, which are important cells of the innate immune response. DCs can be derived from monocytes both in vivo and in vitro, depending on the nature of the cytokines in the environment or in cultures. Also, the functioning of NK cells, which are prominent in the innate immune response, is dependent on the functional state of DCs. In addition, the functioning of natural killer T (NKT) cells may be influenced by DCs. Direct interaction between DCs and NKT cells may be mediated by ligation of CD1d and T-cell receptors. NKT cells can produce both IFN-γ and IL-4 or IL-13.

In addition, it has recently been shown that a subset of DCs is capable of producing type-1 interferon (IFN), which can act as an effector of the innate immune system. Type-1 IFN may also provide the danger signals that induce an adaptive immune response in situ. In addition, DCs produce and induce a variety of cytokines, chemokines, and mediators reflecting their capacity to influence the tissue microenvironment and subsequent adaptive immune responses.

Thus, DCs have the potential to act in both innate and adaptive immune responses. Most importantly, DCs may act as a bridge between these two limbs of the immune system. Plasmacytoid DCs produce IFN-α in vivo in response to microbial infection. This secreted IFN-α in and around the site of microbial infection alters the mucosal milieu and provides the requisite danger signals to myeloid DCs for the induction of adaptive immunity.

DCs can perform a wide variety of the functions of both innate and adaptive immunity owing to their phenotypic and functional diversity. They are endowed with specialized functions from the precursor to the terminally differentiated stages. DC precursors can also induce a variety of immune mediators. Furthermore, DCs are able to polarize T cells to T helper (Th) 1- and Th2-type cells, depending on the dose, affinity, and nature of the antigens and the types and concentrations of cytokines in the tissue microenvironment. The nature of the immune response induced by DCs is also dependent on the DC subtypes that capture the antigens.

The capability of DCs to act in both innate and adaptive immune responses places DCs in a central position in the context of infection with microbial agents. It is the responsibility of DCs to clear the infectious agent by applying all machineries at their disposal. The interactions between DCs and infectious agents primarily determine the successive states of the immune response to the invasive agents, resulting in the clearance or persistence of the infectious agents, or in an abnormal response to them.

DC–Virus Interactions

Introduction

DCs have a dominant role in the induction of the innate immune response, and they also have a pioneering role during the adaptive immune response against infectious agents. After the entry of an infectious agent, as important cells of the innate immune system, DC precursors migrate from the blood to the tissue of viral invasion and produce type-1 IFN and other modulators to destroy the invading virus, in association with other cells of the innate immune system such as macrophages and NK cells. This activity is thought to induce activation of DC precursors or immature DCs in the invaded tissues. These immature DCs recognize the virus or its antigens. Then, DCs capture, process, and present the antigens of the virus to lymphocytes at the immunological synapse in the lymphoid tissues for the induction of adaptive immunity against the virus. DCs also constantly monitor the whole body for the presence of that same virus. When it is detected in any tissues, DCs recognize it and signal antigen-specific lymphocytes to destroy it.

If the interactions of a virus with DCs lead to the induction of the proper innate and virus-specific adaptive immune responses, and if DCs properly interact with other immunocytes in a coordinated manner, the virus should be eradicated from the host. At the same time, the host should be able to prevent any further attack by the same virus owing to the presence of virus-specific memory lymphocytes or specific antibodies.

However, the picture that we observe following infection with viruses varies considerably depending on the nature of the virus and the genetic background and immune status of the host. For example, infection with certain viruses resolves after an acute attack of disease, which is usually self-limiting in nature. However, infections with other viruses become chronic, even in immune-competent hosts. On the other hand, persons infected with some viral infections recover initially, but then relapse, either because of reinfection or owing to a flare-up of infection from hidden sites in the body.

I will discuss our present understanding of virus-DC interactions to develop insights into the pathogenesis of certain viral infections and to evaluate if DCs are involved in the abnormal immune responses observed following some viral infections. I will also summarize some studies on DC-targeting and DC-based therapies for controlling viral infection.

Although the committed function of DCs is to recognize and capture viruses, several reports over the past two decades have provided experimental evidence that DCs from certain virus-infected hosts had impaired functioning, altered phenotypes, immature activation, and defective cytokine production. The viruses that compromise the functional capacities of DCs include hepatitis B virus (HBV), hepatitis C virus (HCV), human immunodeficiency virus (HIV), cytomegalovirus (CMV), Epstein-Barr virus (EBV), measles virus (MV), influenza virus, lymphocytic choriomeningitis virus (LCMV), dengue virus, and several other viruses.

Among these viruses, the interactions of DCs with HIV, MV, and the hepatitis viruses will be discussed in detail.

The interaction of HIV and DCs is interesting because HIV can directly infect DCs. On the other hand, DCs can also capture HIV. Although the infection of DCs by a virus and the capture of a virus by DCs might occur with many viruses, the cellular and molecular mechanisms underlying this phenomenon have been addressed only in HIV. However, the outcome of the DC-HIV interaction does not result in either complete eradication of HIV or the induction of adequate HIV-specific protective immunity.

MV causes direct infection of DCs. This leads to the induction of MV-specific protective immunity as well as to the severe cytopathic destruction of DCs. More importantly, the more severe the destruction of DCs by MV is, the stronger the MV-specific immune responses are in the host.

As these viruses are available in infective form, several in vitro studies have investigated the interactions between them and DCs. Moreover, it is possible to characterize the functioning of DCs from HIV- and MV-infected persons.

It contrast, it is not possible to study the interactions between DCs and hepatitis viruses directly in vitro because infectious virions are not available for such investigations. Different types of hepatitis viruses cause different types of liver diseases. HBV and HCV are the etiological agents of usually progressive, chronic liver diseases, and they cause liver cirrhosis and hepatocellular carcinoma. However, investigations of DC-hepatitis virus interactions have mainly been confined to the characterization of DCs from the infected individuals. Nevertheless, some murine models of chronic infection by hepatitis viruses have provided some important insights into the phenotypes and functions of DCs in chronic carriers of hepatitis viruses. The availability of murine hepatitis virus carriers has also allowed DC-targeting and DC-based therapies to be developed for these chronic hepatitis viral carriers.

Human Immunodeficiency Virus (HIV)

Infection of DCs by HIV

The infection of DCs by HIV and the capture of HIV by DCs will be separately described to gain insight into the DC-virus interactions. One of the most common ways that DCs become infected with HIV is during sexual exposure. Langerhans cells, which are resident DCs in pluristratified epithelia, become infected with HIV. The infection of Langerhans cells and other myeloid DCs by HIV has been known for a quite a long period. Infection of plasmacytoid DCs by HIV has also been reported recently. As DCs are highly mobile, it may be difficult to locate HIV-infected DCs in vivo; they may not be localized at the site of HIV infection. In some experimental models, HIV-infected DCs were not seen in the mucosal tissues after administration of HIV. HIV-infected DCs may be found in the tissue of infection for 18h, but they usually disappear within 48–72h. However, they can be found in lymphoid tissues after 72h, indicating the migration of DCs from the tissue of infection to the lymph nodes after infection with HIV.

The surface expression of CD4 and HIV coreceptors regulates the infection of DCs by HIV. The chemokine receptors CCR5 and CXCR4 are the major HIV coreceptors. HIV can be divided into two types based on the coreceptors required for infection of DCs. R5 viruses (previously termed macrophage-tropic or non-syncytium-inducing viruses) use CCR5 for entry into DCs, whereas HIV types that utilize CXCR4 are termed X4 viruses (previously, T-cell-line-tropic or syncytium-inducing viruses). In general, immature DCs express higher levels of CCR5 and little or no surface CXCR4, whereas mature DCs tend to express less CCR5 and higher levels of CXCR4.

It is now known that R5 viruses are the predominant types transmitted from individual to individual. This type of virus infection is dominant in early stage HIV disease. Naturally, individuals with a homozygous mutation in the open reading frame of *ccr5*, in whom no functional CCR5 protein can be detected, are relatively protected from acquiring HIV despite numerous exposures. As Langerhans cells express CCR5 but not CXCR4, these cells allow R5 infection through mucosa.

Capture of HIV by DCs

Although HIV utilizes CD4 and coreceptors for infecting DCs, several studies in vitro indicate that DCs can also capture HIV by completely different mechanisms. DC-specific intracellular adhesion molecule (ICAM) 3-grabbing nonintegrin (DC-SIGN), a type II membrane protein with an external C-type lectin domain, plays a vital role in the capture of HIV on DCs. DC-SIGN is expressed on the surface of immature and, to a lesser extent, mature DCs. The natural ligands for DC-SIGN are ICAM-3 and ICAM-2. These molecules contribute to the transmigration of DCs across the vascular endothelium. Initially, DC-SIGN was identified by its high-affinity interaction with ICAM-3. Surprisingly, the nucleotide sequence coding for this molecule was found to be identical to that of a previously described HIV glycoprotein (gp) 120-binding C-type lectin gene isolated from a placental cDNA library. DC-SIGN and its homolog (DC-SIGNR) function as attachment factors for HIV-1 and HIV-2. In fact, DC-SIGN affinity for gp120 exceeds that of CD4.

HIV associated with DC-SIGN remains infectious for prolonged periods in the absence of replication within DCs. However, HIV captured by DCs maintains infectivity for 25 days in vitro, whereas free virus rapidly loses its infectious potential.

The mechanisms underlying the prolonged survival of HIV captured by DCs are not well understood. Normally, the capture of a virus by DCs should lead to the internalization of the virus, followed by its degradation. It is curious that DCs cannot digest HIV, and instead protect virions in an infectious form. DC-SIGN is an ICAM-3 receptor with a cytoplasmic domain containing well-defined endocytosis signals. Some investigators have suggested that HIV bound to DC-SIGN, rather than remaining exposed on the surface of DCs, traffics through nonlysosomal endosomal compartments. This would explain why trypsin treatment of HIV-exposed DCs does not decrease the efficacy of DC-mediated virus transmission to T cells.

The Clinical Implications of Infection Versus Capture of HIV by DCs

HIV is transmitted primarily sexually. As HIV can enter DCs by infection, or it can be attached in infectious form by capture, it is important to understand what actually happens following sexual exposure to HIV. The details are unknown, but it is certain that CCR5 plays a vital role in this context. Whether CCR5 influences the initial infection at the immature resident Langerhans cell stage (primary gatekeeper model) or during early replication steps in lymphoid tissue (viral fitness model), or both, however, is less clear. In support of the primary gatekeeper model, recent data indicate that the transmission of the virus from Langerhans cells to T cells is totally dependent on CCR5-mediated infection of Langerhans cells; mannan (which is capable of blocking HIV envelope interactions with C-type lectins), as well as anti-DC-SIGN antibodies, had no effect on Langerhans-cell-mediated transmission of virus to T cells. Furthermore, DC-SIGN might not be involved in the sexual transmission of HIV because it is not expressed by Langerhans cells within the epidermis or vaginal epithelium. Thus, it is likely that CCR5-mediated infection of Langerhans cells, and not DC-SIGN-mediated capture of HIV, is the major pathway of sexual transmission of HIV.

DC-SIGN-mediated capture of HIV by DCs may play a role in the early events of sexual transmission by trapping small amounts of virus produced by Langerhans cells and amplifying viral loads by migrating to lymph nodes and infecting T cells. Indeed, regardless of whether DCs are infected with HIV or hold HIV captured in endosomal compartments, both of these viral states render DCs infectious. Specifically, both HIV-infected DCs and DCs with captured virus transmit robust infection to cocultured $CD4^+$ T cells. Thus, dendritic cell-T cell interactions, critical in the generation of immune responses, also provide rich microenvironments for amplification of HIV replication. In general, the levels of HIV replication in DC-T cell cocultures correlate directly with the degree of T-cell activation in vitro.

In vivo, increases in viral load that are commonly observed during opportunistic infections (e.g., tuberculosis) may be secondary to DC-mediated activation and infection of memory T cells. In this context, we can speculate that DC-SIGN-mediated infection of T cells is the major means by which DCs promote infection of T cells, given that the absolute number of HIV-infected DCs is relatively low in chronically infected individuals. Furthermore, not only does DC-SIGN promote infection of T cells that interact with DCs, this molecule also facilitates the close interaction of HIV gp120 with CD4 and HIV coreceptors on the surfaces of DCs, thus enhancing infection of DCs as well.

In summary, in contrast to sexual transmission of HIV mediated by CD4 and CCR5, DC-SIGN-mediated capture of HIV, with subsequent DC-mediated infection of T cells during the immune response, might contribute greatly to overall viral replication in chronic HIV disease.

DC Dysfunction and Changes in DC Subsets

HIV infection is associated with depletion and dysfunction of DCs. DCs from HIV-infected patients show decreased T-cell stimulatory capacity, which might be related to decreased expression of MHC antigens on DCs. Plasmacytoid DCs may become infected with HIV, and HIV replication may take place in these DCs as well. Viral replication is triggered upon activation of plasmacytoid DCs with CD40L, a signal physiologically delivered by CD4 T cells. Thus, plasmacytoid DCs may play an important role in the dissemination of HIV. These IFN-α-producing DCs directly recognize and respond to HIV-1 with IFN-α production and maturation of DCs. Decreased numbers and decreased functioning of DC subsets (myeloid and plasmacytoid DCs) have been reported in early stage HIV infection. Lower DC numbers may lead to the functional impairment of HIV-specific $CD4^+$ T cells. In HIV carriers, a decrease in the frequency of plasmacytoid DCs and IFN-α production was observed.

Recently, it has been reported that the absolute numbers of myeloid and plasmacytoid DCs in HIV-1-infected subjects were lower than in control subjects, most significantly in those with active HIV-1 replication. Increased surface expression of a costimulatory molecule (CD86) was observed on both DC subsets with HIV-1 viremia.

Therapeutic and Preventive Vaccines for HIV Using DCs

Although HIV-specific immunity wanes in chronically infected individuals, clinical studies have shown that functional immune responses can be augmented following interruptions in highly active antiretroviral therapy. For this reason, HIV researchers have long been interested in immunotherapeutic approaches to HIV disease. DCs, which are the best possible antigen-presenting cells, are good candidate cells for boosting immunity. In vitro, DCs transduced with HIV proteins such as Nef or Gag, or simply pulsed with heat-inactivated viruses or HIV RNA, generate HIV-specific T cells. As well, DCs can process extracellular HIV antigens for presentation by MHC class I molecules in the absence of viral replication; this process, however, requires adequate HIV-surface receptor interactions and fusion of viral and cellular membranes. This "cross-presentation" pathway may play a crucial role in the activation of $CD8^+$ cytotoxic T lymphocytes during viral infections. Monocyte-derived dendritic cells or $CD34^+$ cells that can be expanded and differentiated into DCs can be efficiently transduced using lentiviral vectors. In contrast to retroviral vectors, lentiviral vectors, including HIV- and Simian immunodeficiency virus (SIV)-derived vectors, are able to infect slowly dividing or nondividing cells. When viral vectors are used to transduce DCs, however, the viral mechanisms of immune evasion may paralyze DC functioning. Viral mechanisms that obstruct the generation of antiviral responses are numerous, including interference with the antigen presentation machinery of the infected APC, inhibition of MHC class I, MHC class II, or CD4 expression, interference with transporter associated with antigen processing (TAP) loading mechanisms, and inhibition of dendritic cell maturation. These problems can be circumvented by removing accessory genes that downregulate receptors or antigen presentation.

Numerous strategies are currently being evaluated to develop an AIDS vaccine. In vivo targeting of resident DCs may be the best means to establish a protective primary immune response. In particular, DNA-coated particles injected into skin via gene guns and topical protein patches are vaccine strategies that exploit the immune-stimulating potential of Langerhans cells within the skin. Whether these approaches will elicit better protective immune responses against HIV than more traditional vaccine delivery methods, that is, oral and intramuscular routes, remains to be determined.

Measles Virus

Measles Virus–Dendritic Cell Interactions

Interaction between DCs and measles virus (MV) is a double-edged sword. Infection with MV leads to the development of substantial MV-specific humoral and cellular immune responses, leading to virus clearance and the establishment of a lifelong immunity against reinfection. At the same time, this virus induces severe immuno-suppression. There is a strict correlation between the extent of the MV-specific immune response and the level of immunosuppression.

MV binds to a surface receptor, CD46, one of the regulators of complement activation via hemagglutinin, and then fuses with the cell membrane via its fusion protein. This may lead to the formation of syncytia or multinucleated giant cells (Warthin-Finkeldey cells), which are found in the submucosal regions of the tonsils and pharynx and act as reservoir of MV.

DCs of the respiratory mucosa may be the first target cells to encounter MV during primary infection, and subsequently they transport antigens to the draining lymph nodes to initiate a virus-specific immune response. All types of DCs, including DC progenitors, skin LCs, immature DCs, mature DCs, and activated DCs, can be productively infected with MV at a very low multiplicity of infection. MV-infected DCs also produce infected particles, and some DCs form syncytia. Infection of DCs with MV also influences the viability and integrity of DCs. DCs expressing nucleoprotein undergo apoptosis. When MV-infected DCs are cocultured with activated T cells, MV production in DCs is upregulated and syncytia formation is increased. Finally, both DCs and T cells undergo apoptosis.

Functional Consequences of MV Infection

Downregulation of CD46, an MV receptor, was observed after infection of mature DCs with certain MV strains, whereas expression of specific DC surface markers was not altered. In immature DCs, a rapid maturation, as revealed by the upregulation of HLA-DR, CD40, CD83, CD80, and CD86, was observed after infection, accompanied by the expression of viral glycoproteins.

Conflicting results have been obtained on the release of IL-12 from DCs after MV infection. Whereas MV infection stimulated lipopolysaccharide (LPS)- or *Staphylococcus aureus* Cowan strain (SACS)-induced IL-12 synthesis in one study, a significant inhibition of CD40L-induced IL-12 release has also been described. The impact of MV on IL-12 release from DCs may be dependent on the source or maturation stage of these cells as well as on the strain of MV. In particular, lymphotropic MV wild-type isolates fail to downregulate CD46, and, as shown in recent studies, may not even use this protein as an attachment receptor.

MV-infected DCs largely fail to induce an allostimulatory response when assayed in a mixed leukocyte/lymphocyte reaction (MLR), in spite of their activated phenotype. Moreover, even the mitogen-dependent proliferation of peripheral blood lymphocytes was impaired in the presence of MV-infected DCs. Also, DCs infected with wild-type MV were found to cause stronger suppression, compared with those infected with the vaccine strain of MV. The reasons put forward to explain the loss of allostimulatory properties and the suppressive activities of MV-infected DCs include the loss of both DCs and T cells by apoptosis or cell fusion, depletion of IL-12, and the transfer of MV from DCs to T cells. However, it has been shown experimentally that contact between the MV glycoproteins F and H (on the surfaces of UV-irradiated infected cells, cells transfected with F-H expression constructs, or UV-irradiated viral particles) is sufficient to induce a state of unresponsiveness toward mitogenic, allogenic, or anti-CD3-mediated stimulation in freshly isolated human and rodent peripheral blood lymphocytes (PBLs). Thus, after contact with F-H-expressing cells, PBLs did not undergo apoptosis but rather accumulated in the G1 phase of the cell cycle. Contact-mediated inhibition did not impair the mitogen-induced upregulation of early activation markers, including the IL-2R subunits, and proliferative arrest could not be averted by exogenous IL-2. Thus, since high levels of MV glycoproteins are expressed on the surface of DCs after infection, their inhibitory activity might reflect a dominant negative signaling to T lymphocytes, exerted by MV glycoproteins. In support of this hypothesis, DCs infected with a recombinant MV expressing the vascular stomatitis virus (VSV) G protein, instead of the MV glycoprotein, especially stimulated an MLR and did not inhibit mitogen-dependent proliferation of human PBLs. There may, of course, be additional effects of MV infection on specialized functions of DCs, such as alterations of cytokine reactivity or release, or their ability to capture, process, and present antigens. Mannose receptor-mediated endocytosis, however, was not impaired 2 days after infection of DCs by MV.

MV Interactions with DCs During Natural or Experimental Measles Infection

So far, the role of DCs during natural measles has not been directly assessed. Study of this particular interaction has been hampered by the lack of suitable animal models, as mice and rats cannot be infected by the intranasal route. However, following intranasal infection of juvenile Rhesus monkeys, skin rash, pneumonia, and systemic infection with dissemination to further mucosal sites and to lymphoid tissue was observed. Also, inflammation and necrosis occurred in the lungs and lymphoid tissues, and many cell types, most frequently B cells in lymphoid follicles, were infected with MV after 1 week. MV antigen was found in follicular dendritic cells 14 days after infection. It is unclear whether follicular dendritic cells support virus replication. The impact of infection on bone marrow-derived dendritic cells has not been investigated in this system. The role of DCs during natural measles infection is unknown. Since MV can replicate in DCs generated in vitro, and these cells are comparable to immature DCs, mature interdigitating DCs, and Langerhans cells in vivo, it is likely that natural measles infection is initiated by the uptake and replication of MV within epithelial Langerhans cells and dermal interstitial DCs at mucosal membranes. DCs then migrate to the T-cell areas of lymphoid organs, where they present immunogenic peptides to naive T lymphocytes. This interaction with T cells allows MV to undergo massive replication, to some degree in syncytia, but predominantly in DCs. Once the expression of viral glycoproteins exceeds a certain threshold on the surface of DCs, these cells probably deliver a negative signal to both resting and activated T cells, which contribute to the suppression of T-cell functions directed against opportunistic infections.

Hepatitis Viruses

The interactions between DCs and HIV and MV were studied by directly infecting DCs with the viruses. However, it has not been possible to study such interactions with hepatitis viruses. The dimensions of the problem are also different with different viruses. Both HIV and MV are cytopathic viruses, and infection with these viruses leads to severe opportunistic infection of the host, which is the principle problem in some circumstances. However, infections with hepatitis viruses are not directly cyto-pathic for the infected hosts. Moreover, these viruses do not induce generalized immune suppression. Rather, the immune response of the hosts to the viral or virus-related antigens is responsible for the pathogenic process.

Several hepatitis viruses infect humans and higher primates. Among these, hepatitis A virus and hepatitis E virus cause acute liver inflammation, or the infection may remain masked without any visible symptoms. In either case, infections are usually resolved after an acute attack, although some cases might develop fulminant hepatitis or a severe form of hepatitis with a very bad prognosis.

Infection with HBV or HCV may also cause acute and severe hepatitis. Although understanding the role of DCs in the pathogenesis of severe hepatitis appears to be an interesting and challenging area of clinical immunology, there is little information available. The role of DCs in acute hepatitis has also not been explored because, even though patients with acute hepatitis can transmit viruses, they do not constitute a major public health problem.

DCs have attracted the attention of hepatologists and immunologists in the context of chronic infection by HBV and HCV. For various reasons, some people infected with HBV and HCV cannot clear these viruses, so they become chronic viral carriers. Chronic HBV and HCV infection is also associated with progressive liver diseases, including liver cirrhosis and hepatocellular carcinoma. Epidemiological studies indicate that vertical transmission or infection at an early age underlies the pathogenesis of the chronic HBV carrier state. Recently, evidence has been accumulating that the HBV genotype contributes to persistent HBV infection. On the other hand, infection with HCV can cause chronic infection even when immune-competent adult patients are infected. Some findings of studies on DCs in chronic HBV and HCV infection are summarized in Table 3.1.

Impaired Functioning of DCs in Chronic HBV Carriers

Characterization of DCs in HBV-Transgenic Mice, a Murine Model of the HBV Carrier State. Most studies on DCs in chronic HBV carriers have been done by the research group of F. V. Chisari in the USA or by our group in Japan. HBV carriers are characterized by the presence of HBV and hepatitis B surface antigens (HBsAgs) for more than 6 months. Antibodies to HBsAg (anti-HBs) are the protective antibodies to HBV infection. Development of anti-HBs in HBV carriers indicates the complete cure of chronic HBV infection. Paradoxically, in spite of having high levels of HBsAg, HBV carriers are unable to mount an adequate immune response to HBsAg. When our research group first decided to explore the role of DCs in the pathogenesis of chronic HBV carriers in the early 1990s, there was no methodology to isolate adequate numbers of human DCs for functional studies. Accordingly, we used the HBV-trans-genic (Tg) mouse as an animal model of the HBV carrier state to study the interaction between DCs and HBV. HBV-Tg mice were produced by microinjecting the full genome of HBV into the fertilized eggs of C57BL/6 mice. HBV-Tg mice express HBV virion particles, HBV DNA, HBV-related mRNAs, HBsAgs, and hepatitis B e antigens (HBeAgs) in tissues and sera. In spite of having all HBV-related mRNAs and proteins, the mice did not show any evidence of hepatitis. The absence of hepatitis in HBV-Tg mice provided an added benefit for understanding the interaction between DCs and

Table 3.1. Dendritic cells in chronic HBV and HCV infection

Type of infection and location	Effects
Chronic HBV infection:	
Murine spleen DCs	Low expression of MHC class II, CD86
	Low allostimulatory capacity
	Low production and induction of cytokines
	Decreased stimulation of Ag-specific lymphocytes
Human monocyte-derived peripheral blood DCs	Low allostimulatory capacity
	Low IL-12 production
	Expression of HBV DNA and HBV RNA
DC precursors in the blood	Low allostimulatory capacity
	Low IL-12 production
Chronic HCV infection:	
HCV-transfected spleen DCs	Low allostimulatory capacity
	Low IL-12 production
Human monocyte-derived peripheral blood DCs	Low allostimulatory capacity
	Low IL-12 production
	Infection with HCV RNA
Myeloid DC precursors in blood	Low allostimulatory capacity
	Infected with HCV RNA
	Low IL-12 production
Plasmacytoid DC precursors in blood	Infected with HCV RNA
	Low IFN-α production
	Decreased myeloid DCs
	Decreased polarization to Th1

HBV because factors related to hepatitis could not influence the functioning of DCs in this animal model.

Similar to patients with chronic HBV infection, HBV-Tg mice were also unable to respond to HBsAg, and anti-HBs were not detected in the sera in any HBV-Tg mice in our study. HBV-Tg mice also did not show any cellular immune response to HBsAg.

As HBV-Tg mice harbored intrauterine-acquired HBsAg, it is possible that HBsAg is a tolerogen in HBV-Tg mice. To test this, we checked the immune response of HBV-Tg mice to keyhole limpet hemocyanin (KLH), an HBV-unrelated, T-cell-dependent antigen. To our surprise, we found that the cellular and humoral immune responses of HBV-Tg mice to KLH were also impaired. A series of coculture experiments showed that the functional impairment of spleen DCs was responsible for the defective immune response of HBV-Tg mice to KLH. The impaired APC functioning of spleen DCs from HBV-Tg mice was due to their low expression of MHC class II antigens and CD86. DCs from HBV-Tg mice were also poor inducers and producers of proinflammatory cytokines such as IL-12, TNF-α, and IFN-γ.

The impaired immune response of HBV-Tg mice to HBsAg is understandable, but the mechanism of the impaired immune response to KLH is hard to explain. It indicates a very specific defect of the antigen presentation capacity of DCs of these mice to T-cell-dependent Ags. Several viruses are known to compromise the functioning of DCs or other immunocytes by producing inhibitory proteins, inducing apoptosis, depleting DCs, or by some other unknown mechanisms. The exact causes underlying the impaired KLH-specific immune response in HBV-Tg mice are still elusive. However, as HBV and its products had been circulating in HBV-Tg mice, HBV-related factors are the most likely candidates to explain the impaired DC functioning in these mice.

Functional Impairment of DCs from Patients with Chronic Hepatitis B. In the meantime, DCs were enriched from patients with chronic hepatitis B (CH-B) and studied their functioning and checked whether they were harboring HBV DNA or RNA. Using the polymerase chain reaction (PCR) and reverse transcriptase PCR in situ hybridization methods, we showed that 20%–40% of DCs from CH-B patients were harboring HBV DNA and RNA (Fig. 3.1). Functionally, the allostimulatory capacities of DCs from CH-B patients were significantly lower than those of normal controls or patients with nonviral chronic hepatitis. DCs from these patients also produced and induced significantly lower levels of IL-12 in DC-T cell cultures compared with controls. Two independent laboratories that enriched DCs from two different ethnic groups also reported impaired function of DCs from CH-B patients. Further evidence of the contribution of DCs to the pathogenesis of CH-B was provided when a disproportional distribution of plasmacytoid and myeloid DCs were reported in CH-B patients. Increased frequencies of plasmacytoid DCs, decreased numbers of myeloid DCs, and functional impairment of myeloid DCs from CH-B patients were reported. Plasmacytoid DCs are known to produce type-I IFN in vitro as a result of viral stimulation, but they also induce Th2 polarization, whereas myeloid DCs induce Th1 polarization. The increased polarization to a Th2 phenotype in CH-B patients might be related to the inability of CH-B patients to clear HBV. However, it will be important to evaluate the levels of type-1 IFN production by plasmacytoid DCs from CH-B patients.

These studies in HBV-Tg mice and in patients with CH-B indicate that infection, dysfunction, and an abnormal distribution of DCs are characteristic of chronic HBV infection. However, the following aspects of DC involvement in chronic HBV infection must be understood before DCs can be brought from the lab bench to the bedside of CH-B patients.

1. The most important issue is the recognition of HBsAg by tissue DCs in chronic HBV carriers (liver DCs, in this case). HBsAg may behave like a self-antigen in chronic HBV carriers. Again, HBV and HBsAg may not provide adequate danger signals for DC mobilization in these patients. It is important to evaluate whether DCs mobilize to the liver after HBV infection. The liver harbors DC progenitors, which are mostly tolerogenic in nature. How liver DC progenitors alter their phenotype and function after HBV infection is important in this regard. Although these are important points, in many people HBV infection is a self-limiting or self-resolving infection. What are the fundamental differences between acutely infected and chronically infected patients. The migratory capacity of DCs from the liver to the regional lymph nodes might be important. The impaired functioning of spleen DCs in HBV-Tg mice may reflect a generalized defect in the functioning of DCs in these mice. However, the recognition, mobilization, capture, processing, migration, and presentation of HBV by DCs in the animal model of the HBV carrier state must be studied, although methodologies to check many of these cellular events have not yet been developed.

2. The characterization of the functioning of different subsets of DCs in CH-B patients is most important. Patients with CH-B follow a chronic pathological course

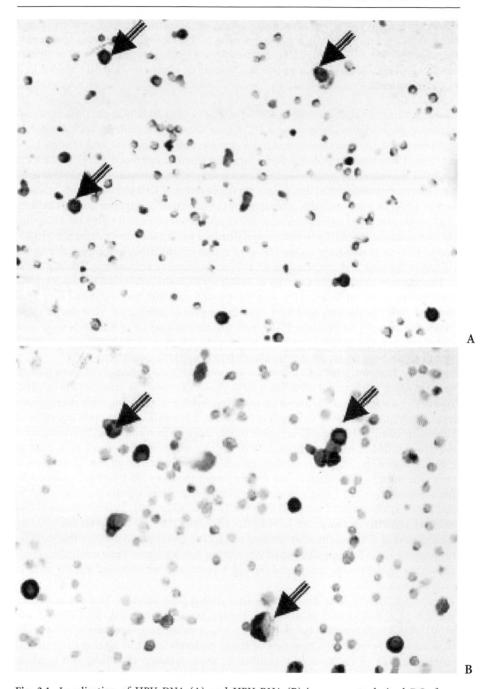

Fig. 3.1. Localization of HBV DNA (**A**) and HBV RNA (**B**) in monocyte-derived DCs from patients with chronic hepatitis B. Signals for HBV DNA and HBV RNA were detected as blackish (*arrow head*) by in situ polymerase chain reaction (PCR) hybridization, and reverse transcriptase (RT)-PCR hybridization. Signals for HBV DNA and HBV RNA were detected in 20%–40% of DCs from patients with chronic hepatitis B. Original magnification ×300

characterized by exacerbation and remission of hepatitis. Several cytokines and chemokines are differentially regulated during this pathological process. Apparently, the allostimulatory function of DCs can be affected by the action of several cytokines in vivo. It is necessary to evaluate the functioning of plasmacytoid and myeloid DCs in CH-B patients.

Upregulation of DC Functioning in HBV-Tg Mice In Vivo by Polyclonal Immune Modulator: A First Step in Developing a DC-Based Therapy for Patients with CH-B. As impairment of DC functioning has been demonstrated in murine and human HBV carriers, it has been postulated that a new therapeutic approach for HBV carriers might be developed by improving the functioning of DCs in vivo. To attain this goal, our laboratory attempted to upregulate the functioning of DCs in vivo by IFN-γ. Injection of HBV-Tg mice with IFN-γ resulted in (1) increased T-cell stimulatory capacity of DCs; (2) increased expression of MHC class II molecules and CD86 on DCs; and (3) increased ability of DCs to induce and produce proinflammatory cytokines. Injection of IFN-γ was also accompanied by a reduction in HBV DNA in the liver, decreased HBsAg in the sera, and an increased KLH-specific immune response in HBV-Tg mice.

The immune modulatory capacity of IFN-γ on DCs was confirmed by checking the functioning of spleen DCs in IFN-γ Tg mice and found that they exhibited very high levels of IFN-γ in the sera and liver. The expression of MHC class II molecules and CD86, the capacity to produce IL-12, and the functioning of spleen DCs were also highly exacerbated in IFN-γ Tg mice compared with normal mice. DCs from IFN-γ Tg mice also induced a potent immune response to T cell-dependent Ag.

Ag-Specific Stimulation of DCs (Vaccine Therapy) in HBV-Tg Mice. Next, even though we were using a polyclonal modulator (IFN-γ), we attempted to activate DCs in HBV-Tg mice in an Ag-specific manner by injecting HBsAg in adjuvant. This therapy was termed vaccine therapy as HBsAg is also used in a prophylactic vaccine. Injection of HBsAg in complete Freund's adjuvant (CFA) once each month for 12 consecutive months resulted in complete negativity of HBsAg and HBeAg in about 60%–80% of HBV-Tg mice (Fig. 3.2). This serological effect of the vaccination was accompanied by a reduction in HBV DNA in the sera by more than 10–100 times (as assessed by semi-quantitative PCR) and a more than 80% reduction in signals for HBV DNA in the liver (as determined by in situ hybridization) (Fig. 3.3). Vaccine therapy also induced anti-HBs in about 25% of HBV-Tg mice. The HBV-Tg mice were followed up for a period of 3–6 months after the end of vaccine therapy, and none of the vaccine-responding HBV-Tg mice developed circulating HBsAg again. Four controlled trials of vaccine therapy were conducted during 4 years, and we obtained similar data in each of these trials.

Therapy for HBV-Tg Mice by Targeting DCs with a DNA Vaccine. Two plasmid DNA vectors, pCAGGS(S) and pCAGGS (S+preS2), were constructed. pCAGGS(S) and pCAGGS (S+preS2) contain the genes of the major envelope and middle envelope proteins of HBV, respectively. Injection of these plasmids into the regenerating tibialis anterior muscle of C57BL/6 mice resulted in the expression of HBsAg and localization of CD11c+ DCs in the HBV-Tg mice (Fig. 3.4). Injection of DNA vaccines resulted in expression of HBsAg in immunogenic form in spleen DCs from HBV-Tg mice. A single injection of DNA vaccine cleared HBsAg and HBeAg from more than 90% of HBV-Tg mice and induced production of anti-HBs in about 50% of them.

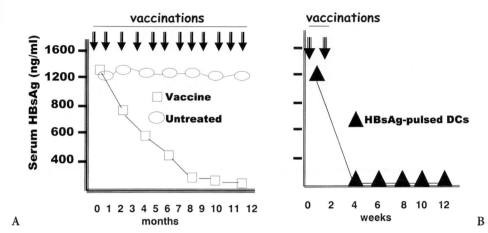

Fig. 3.2A,B. Therapeutic response of vaccine therapy targeting DCs or DC-based immune therapy in HBV-transgenic (Tg) mouse. There was a slow and gradual decrease in hepatitis B surface antigen (HBsAg) in HBV-Tg mice as a result of 12 monthly vaccinations with commercial vaccine (*squares*). However, untreated HBV-Tg mice (*circles*) did not show any decrease (A). In contrast, HBV-Tg mice injected only twice with HBsAg-pulsed DCs (*solid triangles*) 2 weeks apart, cleared HBsAg from HBV-Tg mice within 4 weeks

Vaccine Therapy Targeting DCs in Patients with CH-B. After conducting vaccine therapy in HBV-Tg mice, we tested it in CH-B patients. The CH-B patients received 20 µg of HBsAg once every 2 weeks for 24 weeks (12 doses). The vaccine therapy was uneventful; about two thirds of the patients responded to vaccine therapy by showing normalization of transaminases and reduced replication of HBV DNA. The activation of DC maturation by the vaccine therapy was responsible for its therapeutic effect (Fig. 3.5).

In some viral infections, such as MV infection, the degree of functional impairment of DCs depends on viral load and antigen load. Accordingly, we speculated that if HBV could be reduced by antiviral therapy, that might prepare the way for the action of vaccine therapy. A group of CH-B patients was first given lamivudine, an antiviral agent, for 3 months and then 12 doses of vaccine therapy. Another group of patients received only lamivudine therapy. All patients receiving both lamivudine and vaccine became negative for HBV DNA (*n* = 15), whereas fewer than half of the patients receiving only lamivudine became negative for HBV DNA. A study of DC functioning in these groups of patients provided very interesting information. The allostimulatory capacities of DCs in the patients with CH-B were significantly lower compared with control subjects. When these patients were treated with lamivudine, DC functioning was increased. When they were treated with vaccine after 3 months of lamivudine therapy, DC functioning was further elevated and remained so as long as the vaccine therapy was continued.

DC-Based Vaccine for Chronic HBV Carriers. Activation of DCs by vaccines was responsible for the therapeutic effect of vaccine therapy in HBV-Tg mice and in CH-B patients. On the other hand, although vaccine therapy seemed to be a potent

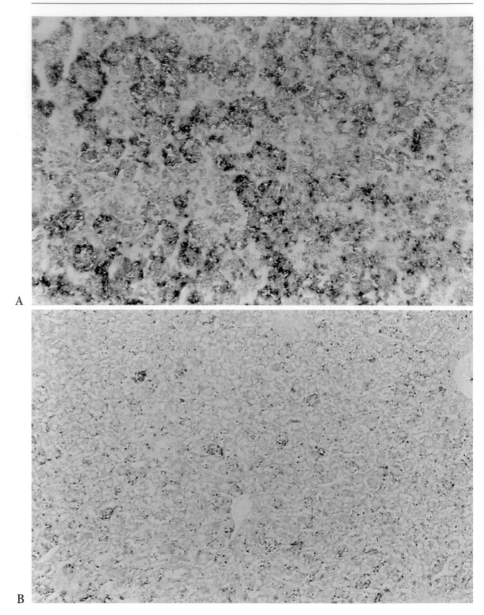

Fig. 3.3. The antiviral potential of vaccine therapy targeting DCs in HBV-Tg mice. Decreased HBV DNA in the liver due to vaccine therapy in HBV-Tg mice: HBV DNA was localized in the liver by in situ hybridization using a HBV DNA-specific probe. **A** The signals for HBV DNA in untreated HBV-Tg mice. **B** The signals for HBV DNA reduced drastically after 12 months of vaccine therapy. Original magnification ×110. HBV DNA is shown by *black signals*

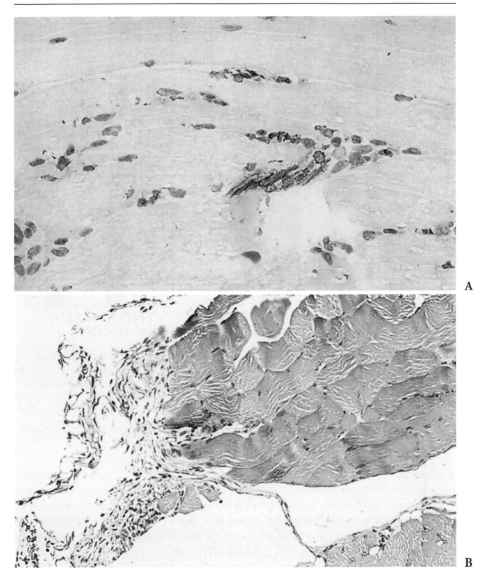

Fig. 3.4A,B. Localization of DCs and expression of proteins in muscles after injecting plasmids encoding the DNA vaccines. Seventy-two hours after injection of DNA vaccine containing plasmid encoding DNA of hepatitis B surface antigen (HBsAg), CD11c⁺ DCs localized at the site of injection (**A**). Original magnification ×450. HBsAg was also expressed at the site of DNA vaccination (**B**). Original magnification ×225. Positive signals for DCs and HBsAg are shown by *bluish staining*

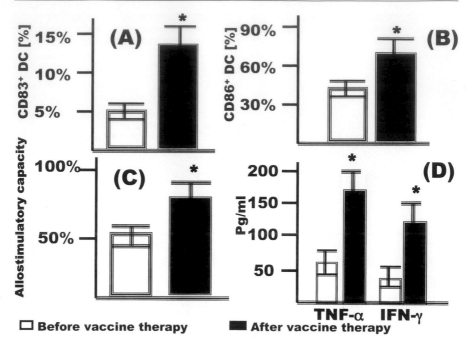

Fig. 3.5A–D. Upregulation of the functions of peripheral blood DCs after vaccine therapy in patients with chronic hepatitis B (CH-B). The numbers of CD83+ DCs (**A**), and CD86+ DCs (**B**) among bulk populations of DCs increased significantly after vaccine therapy in patients with CH-B (*black*) compared to their pre-vaccinated levels (*white*). The allostimulatory capacity of DCs (**C**) and the production of cytokines by DCs (**D**) also increased after vaccine therapy (*black*) compared with before (*white*) the start of vaccine therapy. *$P < 0.05$

immune therapy for HBV carriers, it had two major limitations. One was its inability to induce anti-HBs in 100% of HBV-Tg mice, and the other was its inability to clear HBsAg in any patients with CH-B. To develop a more potent therapeutic vaccine for HBV carriers, we loaded HBsAg on spleen DCs from HBV-Tg mice, confirmed the pulsing of DCs with HBsAg, and then injected these HBsAg-loaded DCs into HBV-Tg mice twice, 2 weeks apart (Fig. 3.2B). All HBV-Tg mice receiving these HBsAg-pulsed DCs became negative for HBsAgs and developed anti-HBs.

DCs in Chronic HCV Infection

Because of the absence of proper animal models for the HCV carrier state expressing the full genome of HCV, we studied DC functioning by transfecting spleen DCs from normal C57BL/6 mice with adenovirus vector containing the HCV gene. Spleen DCs expressing HCV antigens showed impaired allostimulatory function and low IL-12 production, indicating that HCV also affects the functioning of DCs. Further study revealed that the expression of HCV-related proteins led to impaired transmission of intracellular peptides. Moreover, the expression of MHC class I and class II antigens was distorted by transfection with HCV.

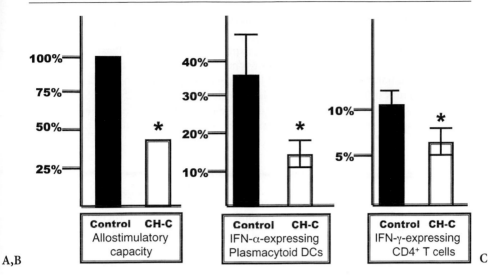

A,B   C

Fig. 3.6A–C. Impaired function of circulatory DCs in patients with CH-C. Bulk populations of circulatory DCs containing both myeloid and plasmacytoid DCs were isolated by magnetic cell sorting. Circulatory DCs were detected as lineage⁻, CD4⁺, HLA DR⁺ cells of the peripheral blood mononuclear cells (PBMCs). Plasmacytoid DCs were identified as lineage⁻, HLA DR⁺, CD11c⁻, and CD123⁺ cells among the bulk population of DCs. A The mean allostimulatory capacity of DCs from 20 normal control is shown as 100%. The mean allostimulatory capacity of DCs from CH-C patients was 35% of that of controls. B Stimulation with herpes simplex virus-1 resulted in the production of intracellular IFN-α in plasmacytoid DCs. The frequency of IFN-α-producing plasmacytoid DCs was significantly lower in patients with chronic C than in controls. C Naive CD4⁺ T cells were stimulated by DCs for 7 days and the frequency of CD4⁺ T cells expressing IFN-γ was determined by flow cytometry. *$P < 0.05$ compared with normal controls

In patients with chronic hepatitis C (CH-C), the functioning of DCs has been studied by various groups, including ours (Table 3.1). In most of these studies, DCs were enriched from peripheral blood mononuclear cells by culturing them with a cocktail of cytokines. The allostimulatory capacity of DCs was significantly decreased in patients with CH-C compared with controls (Fig. 3.6). DCs from CH-C patients produced less IL-12, and they also supported the replication of HCV, as was evident from the presence of minus-strand HCV RNA in DCs. DCs from CH-C patients could not adequately activate NK cells in response to IFN-α stimulation, probably as a result of decreased expression of MHC class 1-related chains A and B (MICA/B) on DCs.

Recently, we isolated circulating DCs from peripheral blood of CH-C patients by using cell-sorting techniques. The functioning of circulating DCs was also significantly lower compared with that of normal controls. HCV RNA was detected in bulk populations of circulating DCs as well as in plasmacytoid and myeloid DCs. Therapy of CH-C patients with antiviral agents such as ribavirin restored the functioning of the DCs.

Type-1 IFN-Producing Plasmacytoid DCs. Plasmacytoid DCs, which are recognized in the peripheral blood by their lineage negativity, CD11c negativity, and expression of

CD4 and CD123, are a precursor population of DCs. These cells are also called pDC2 and lymphoid DCs. They lack a potent antigen-capturing apparatus but can migrate directly to lymphoid tissues owing to their expression of L-selectin. Plasmacytoid DCs are able to produce abundant amounts of type-1 IFN in response to some viruses. A study in our laboratory has shown that the capacity of plasmacytoid DCs to produce IFN-α is significantly decreased in patients with CH-C compared with control subjects (Fig. 3.6). Moreover, the frequency of myeloid DCs decreased, and these DCs had impaired capacity to induce Th1 polarization compared with DCs of the controls (Fig. 3.6).

Chemokines and DCs in Patients with Chronic Hepatitis

The migratory property of DCs is unique because owing to this capacity, DCs are able to mobilize in the tissue and migrate to lymph nodes after antigen processing. Expression of chemokine receptors on DCs and chemokines in target organs is essential for their migratory capacity in vivo. Immature DCs express CCR6 and migrate in response to the chemokine macrophage inflammatory protein (MIP) 3α, whereas mature DCs express CCR7, which moves to MIP-3β and SLC. The expression of MIP-3α at the site of the hepatitis interface in patients with chronic hepatitis indicates that migration of immature DCs might be retained in patients with chronic hepatitis. The serum levels of MIP-3α were checked in these patients, and the levels of this chemokine were increased in the sera of patients with chronic hepatitis. Although, the relationship between this chemokine and its receptor in DCs has not been checked, the high levels of this chemokine may account for the persistence of immature DCs in hepatitis.

Altered DC Functioning and Phenotypes in the Liver in Hepatitis

Information is accumulating regarding spleen DCs in HBV-Tg mice and blood DCs and DC precursors in CH-B patients, but these DCs are not directly related to the APC functions of DCs, although they may play a potent role in immune therapy. Three DC-related antibodies were used to detect DCs from liver of patients with CH-B and CH-C. These were antibodies to HLA DR, interdigitating dendritic cell (IDC), S100, and CD83 antigens. To identify the CD83 antigen, we employed an antigen retrieval technique. Many HLA DR-positive cells are located in and around the hepatitis interface and also in the hepatic parenchyma of liver specimens from patients with CH-B and CH-C. IDC- and S100-positive DCs or DC-like cells were also found in liver specimens from these patients. CD83-positive DCs, although few, were seen in the liver specimens.

DCs were isolated from liver specimens collected during surgery and checked the proportions of plasmacytoid and myeloid DCs among the liver-infiltrating DCs. The numbers of plasmacytoid DCs were about three times those in the blood, indicating that these cells may be localized preferentially in the liver during chronic hepatitis. However, it was not possible to study the functional capacity of liver DCs owing to technical limitations.

To investigate this phenomenon, we established an animal model of hepatitis by injecting concanavalin (Con)-A into C57BL/6 mice. Liver DCs were isolated at the peak of hepatitis. Liver DCs from these mice had a low capacity to present HBsAgs and to induce cytokines from HBsAg-specific memory lymphocytes. This study showed that liver DCs are immunogenic in the context of the presentation of specific antigens. Kupffer cells in liver have been reported to induce immune tolerance to environmental and dietary antigens. A working partnership between immunogenic DCs and tolerogenic Kupffer cells might be important for the maintenance of homeostasis.

Concluding Remarks

As professional APCs, DCs are assumed to play a role in the induction, progression, and complications of chronic infection with hepatitis virus. However, the interaction of HBV and HCV with DCs cannot be studied directly. Available scientific methodologies allowed us to explore the nature of the defects of DCs in chronic HBV and HCV carriers. Those studies showed defective functioning, infection, and deregulation of spleen DCs in HBV-Tg mice and of blood DCs in patients with chronic hepatitis B and C. Impaired functioning of liver DCs in the murine model of acute hepatitis has been reported by only one study. It is necessary to understand the involvement of DCs in the pathogenesis of acute hepatitis and chronic hepatitis. Is it a result of defective recognition of HBV- and HCV-related Ags by liver DCs or of the defective capacity of Ag-bearing DCs to activate T cells in the secondary lymph nodes? The effect of viral factors on DC migration may also be important.

However, in spite of all these limitations, immune therapy targeting DCs or DC-based immune therapy have shown favorable outcomes in murine and human HBV carriers without any apparent side effects. As plasmacytoid DCs produce IFN-α, new therapeutic measures will be developed to upregulate the endogenous production of IFN-α by plasmacytoid DCs in these patients. HBsAg-pulsed DCs have shown dramatic therapeutic potential in HBV-Tg mice, but their effectiveness in CH-B patients is yet to be evaluated.

Although impaired functioning of DCs has been shown in CH-C patients, DC-based therapy or DC-targeting therapy has not been attempted. The major limitation of using such therapies in CH-C patients is the lack of a proper antigen of HCV.

Other Viruses

In addition to HIV, MV, and hepatitis viruses, interactions between DCs and other viruses have been studied by several investigators. DCs support the replication of CMV. Virus replication is observed in CD14$^+$, CD1a$^+$, CD83$^+$ mature DCs, but not in immature myeloid DCs induced by IL-4 and GM-CSF. Thus, peripheral blood mononuclear cells (PBMCs) may harbor latent human CMV, which reactivates in a myeloid lineage cell upon allogenic stimulation. These data suggest that CMV latently infects pro-myeloid DCs and is reactivated in differentiated DCs or macrophages.

Influenza virus infects DCs, and viral proteins such as HA and NS1 proteins are expressed on DCs, but the replication of this virus is not so pronounced in DCs compared with other viruses. Encounters of DCs with influenza virus cause DC maturation, as shown by the expression of DC-LAMP and CD83. Expression of MHC class I and MxA proteins is also seen in influenza-infected DCs. MxA production might help DCs escape from injury by the influenza virus. Thus, DC activation results not only in increased antigen presentation and T-cell stimulatory capacity with up-regulation of MHC, adhesion, and costimulatory molecules, but also in resistance to the cytopathic effect of the virus, mediated by the production of type-1 IFN and upregulation of MxA protein. Cross-priming in influenza virus infection has been studied experimentally. Monocytes infected by influenza virus underwent apoptosis, and immature DCs phagocytose this apoptotic product and induce influenza virus-specific, MHC class I-restricted CD8$^+$ cytotoxic T lymphocytes (CTLs). Phago-cytosis was observed in 80% of macrophages, 50% of immature DCs, and less than 10% of mature DCs. However, CTL activity by cross-priming is most potent in imma-ture DCs and absent in macrophages. Thus, DCs use unique pathways for phagocy-tosis, processing, and presentation of antigens derived from apoptotic cells on MHC class I molecules. CD36 might be important in this cross-priming system. In general, myeloid DCs can polarize T cells toward Th1, and plasmacytoid DCs produce type-1 IFN and polarize T cells toward Th2. However, in presence of influenza virus and CD40L in vitro, plasmacytoid DCs may also polarize to Th1 with upregulation of MHC proteins and costimulatory molecules. Plasmacytoid DCs probably participate in antiviral and proinflammatory responses, as well as Th2 polarization and tolerance induction.

Bacterial Infection

Introduction

DCs have a privileged distribution in tissues that interface with the external environ-ment and therefore can act as proper sentinels against invading bacteria. However, both bacterial cells and DCs have a net negative charge. Thus, specific molecular inter-actions, including bridging molecules, are involved in the uptake of bacteria by DCs. Bacteria such as bacillus Calmette-Guerin, *Saccharomyces aureus, Corynebacterium parvum, Staphylococcus aureus*, and *Borrelia burgdorferi* have been shown to be inter-nalized by DCs, especially immature DCs. The cellular mechanism of internalization of bacteria by DCs may differ depending on the involvement of Fc receptors or complement receptors. Bacterial pseudopodia are involved when Fc receptors of DCs function in the internalization of bacteria. DCs may use macropinocytosis and coiling phagocytosis simultaneously with conventional phagocytosis for the uptake of bacteria.

DCs use different methods for internalization of bacteria, perhaps because of the nature of the bacteria, but different types of immune responses may be initiated by the different internalization methods as well. Thus, different internalization methods may have functional implications. Internalization of bacteria by DCs may take place by nonopsonic uptake, that is, by direct interaction between microbial adhesions and phagocytic receptors, or by opsonic uptake, during which antibodies or complements act as bridging molecules between the microbial surface and opsonin receptors of the DC. Fc receptors, mannose receptors, and Toll-like receptors (TLRs) on DCs and LPS, lipoteichoic acid, and peptidoglycans on the bacteria participate in the recognition and internalization of bacteria by DCs.

After infection of DCs with bacteria, production of cytokines such as TNF-α and IL-6 increases. This is true with both Gram-positive and Gram-negative bacteria. DCs are usually activated by living bacteria. Heat-inactivated bacteria induce phenotypical maturation of DCs, but without cytokine production. IL-12 is produced by DCs under bacterial stimulation. IL-10, which modulates DC growth by inducing the downregulation of CD1, might convert DCs into macrophage-like cells, thereby inhibiting the growth of an intracellular pathogen. Granuloma formation is seen after infection by certain bacteria. Various types of DCs have been found in granulomas, but the role of DCs in their formation remains to be studied.

Mycobacterium tuberculosis

The interaction between *Mycobacterium tuberculosis* and DCs has been well studied. *Mycobacterium tuberculosis* is phagocytosed by both macrophages and DCs. One of the modes of entry of *Mycobacterium tuberculosis* into DCs is via DC-SIGN, which is likely to influence bacterial persistence and host immunity. Immature DCs are found in lung. The expression of MHC class I and II, CD40, ICAM-1 antigens is elevated in *Mycobacterium tuberculosis*-infected DCs. However, infected monocytes do not exhibit enhanced costimulatory or MHC class I molecule expression. The infected DCs produce TNF-α, IL-1, and IL-12 and become mature DCs. On the other hand, phagocytic activity is decreased by infection. IFN-γ, a Th1 cytokine, is an important factor in host defense immunity against *Mycobacterium tuberculosis* infection. On the other hand, Th2 cytokines seems to have no direct effect against *Mycobacterium tuberculosis* infection, according to a study of IL-4, IL-5, and IL-10 knockout mice. Thus, Th2 cytokines are not essential for and do not negatively influence the protective immune response against *Mycobacterium tuberculosis*. However, IFN-γ and IL-2 in sera is elevated in the early stage of *Mycobacterium tuberculosis* infection, and IL-4 and IL-10 is elevated in sera in late stages of the infection. These data suggest that Th2 cytokines affect the progression of disease and explain the finding that early tuberculosis is characterized by preserved cellular immune responses, whereas the advanced disease is accompanied by their impairment. *Mycobacterium tuberculosis* infection activates cellular immunity. Induction of Th1 cells and production of IFN-γ is important to prevent the progression of disease. In early stages of *Mycobacterium tuberculosis* infection, the presence of cells of the innate immune system, such as macrophages, in the lung is important.

Mature DCs migrate to lymph nodes and activate T cells. DCs produce IL-12, which facilitates the Th1 dominant response. *Mycobacterium tuberculosis* antigen has many lipids on the cell surface. Specific *Mycobacterium tuberculosis* lipids such as mycolic acid and lipoarabinomannan (LAM) are presented to T cells via a CD1 molecule. The purified CD1b-restricted antigen of *Mycobacterium tuberculosis* presented to alpha beta TCR+ T cells is mycolic acid. CD1-restricted antigen presentation does not require any other molecule; MHC-restricted antigen presentation require TAP or HLA-DM.

DC-SIGN, upon the binding of man-LAM, interferes with TLR-mediated signals. Thus, *Mycobacterium tuberculosis* targets DC-SIGN both to infect DCs and to downregulate DC-mediated immune responses.

Mycobacterium tuberculosis induces IL-10 production and suppresses the production of IL-12 in macrophages. IL-10 not only suppresses the replication of *Mycobacterium tuberculosis* in immature DCs but also decreases the T-cell proliferation activity of DCs and their expression of MHC class II molecules. This effect of IL-10 can be overcome by IFN-γ priming.

On the other hand, infected immature DCs show elevated expression of CD14 and elevated phagocytic activity. Thus, *Mycobacterium tuberculosis* infection changes immature DCs to macrophage-like cells. In peripheral blood, the number of myeloid DCs (DC1) was decreased compared with normal controls. In tissue (lung), many myeloid DCs were observed in the lymphocyte areas of tuberculous granulomas (tubercles). IFN-γ-producing Th1 cells also became more numerous. These data suggest that the trafficking of DCs from the peripheral blood into the tubercles causes Th1 dominance and thus plays an essential role in tuberculosis immunity.

Salmonella typhimurium

Salmonella is a Gram-negative bacterium that infiltrates the epithelial barrier of the small intestine. In the small intestine, villi on the surface of epithelial cells and tight junctions between epithelial cells are the barriers against bacterial invasion. M cells overlying the lymphoid follicles of Peyer's patches are important, but they are not the only cells in this mucosal defensive immune system. M cells might provide a portal of entry for pathogens such as *Salmonella typhimurium*. CD18 is a leukocyte adhesion molecule expressed on macrophages and DCs. Both CD18$^+$ macrophages and DCs are found in Peyer's patches and might participate in the capture of *Salmonella* in the intestinal tract. However, *Salmonella* is transported from the gastrointestinal tract to the blood stream by CD18$^-$ phagocytes. CD18-deficient mice are resistant to the dissemination of *Salmonella* to the liver and spleen after oral administration of the pathogen.

In addition, it has been reported that DCs open the tight junctions between epithelial cells, send dendrites outside the epithelium, and directly sample bacteria. Because DCs express tight-junction proteins such as occluding, claudin 1, and zonula occludens 1, the integrity of the epithelial barrier is preserved.

Besides the transport of *Salmonella* across the intestinal barrier, changes in the number, localization, and cytokine production of CD8α^+, VD8α^-, CD4$^+$ and CD8α^-, CD4$^-$ DC subsets occur during *Salmonella* infection. DCs stimulate bacterium-specific T cells by direct presentation of *Salmonella* antigens and bystander APCs. DC cytokine production capacity, particularly of the CD8α+, VD8α^-, CD4$^+$ and CD8α^-, CD4$^-$ DC subsets, was examined. TNF-α was produced by a large percentage of CD8α^- DCs, whereas the greatest numbers of IL-12 p40-producing DCs were CD8α^+ DCs. Thus, DCs in sites of *Salmonella* replication and T-cell activation, spleen and mesenteric lymph nodes, respond to bacterial encounters by antigen presentation and produce cytokines in a subset-specific manner.

Parasitic Infections

Malaria

The malaria parasite (*Plasmodium falciparum*) invades the human body via mosquito bites. After replication in the liver, the malaria parasite is released into the blood, where it infects red blood corpuscles (RBCs). Infected RBCs bind to vascular epithelial cells, platelets, uninfected RBCs, macrophages, and myeloid DCs. *Plasmodium falciparum* malaria is characterized by poor induction of a long-lasting protective immune response.

Infected RBCs bind to DCs via CD36 and CD51 on DCs. Binding suppresses not only the maturation of the DCs (by suppression of MHC class II, ICAM-1, CD83, and CD86 on the surface of the DC) but also the activation of T cells by the DCs. Furthermore, it suppresses the production of IL-12 and enhances the production of IL-10. Thus, intact malaria-infected RBCs adhere to DCs, inhibit their maturation, and consequently reduce their capacity to stimulate T cells.

The percentage of HLA-DR$^+$ peripheral blood DCs is significantly reduced in children with malaria. These data suggest that a proportion of peripheral blood DCs may be functionally impaired by low expression of HLA-DR on their surfaces. For protection against malaria, a CD8$^+$ T-cell response is needed.

Leishmania

Leishmaniasis, a vector-borne parasitic disease, is transmitted during a sand fly blood meal when the parasite is delivered into the dermis. *Leishmania* infects macrophages and DCs. DC-SIGN expressed on DCs is a receptor for *Leishmania* amastigotes. The blocking monoclonal antibody dramatically reduces internalization of *Leishmania* amastigotes by immature DCs.

DCs take up *Leishmania major* and, after it is internalized, undergo changes in surface phenotype suggesting maturation. Infected DCs produce IL-12, which is important for inducing a Th1-type immune response. This IL-12 production depends on the CD40-CD40 ligand interaction. The activation of Th1 followed by IL-12 production by DCs is important to eliminate *Leishmania*. However, in *Leishmania amazonensis* infection in easily infectable mice (BALB/c mice), DCs produce IL-4 rather than IL-12 and induce a Th2-type response. These data suggest that *Leishmania amazonensis* amastigotes may condition DCs of a susceptible host to a state that favors activation of pathogenic CD4$^+$ T cells.

DCs from mice with a chronic *Leishmania donovani* infection fail to migrate from the marginal zone to the periarteriolar region of the spleen. Defective localization was attributed to TNF-α-dependent, IL-10-mediated inhibition of CCR7 expression. The defective DC migration plays a major role in the pathogenesis of leishmaniasis, and the immunosuppression is mediated, at least in part, by the spatial segregation of DCs and T cells.

Toxoplasma

Toxoplasma gondii is an obligate intracellular parasite. It infects a wide variety of nucleated cells of intermediate hosts. IFN-γ activation inhibits the replication of *Toxoplasma gondii* in DCs. DCs may act as effector cells of the early defense mechanism. Induction of chemokines by invading *Toxoplasma gondii* is important not only for the recruitment of DCs but also for the determination of their subsequent immunology function.

TLRs are suggested to play a role in the activation of DCs. The effects of TLR-4, TLR-2, and myeloid differentiation marker 88 (MyD88) were compared between *Tox-*

oplasma gondii-infected wild-type mice and mice deficient in these molecules. MyD88-deficient mice died, whereas TLR-4- and TLR-2-deficient mice survived an intraperitoneal infection by *Toxoplasma gondii*. In MyD88-deficient mice, a high *Toxoplasma gondii* load was observed in the brain, liver, and other organs.

Recommended Readings

Akbar SMF, Horiike N, Onji M, Hino O (2001) Dendritic cells and chronic hepatitis viral carriers. Intervirology 44:199–208

Bhardwaj N (1997) Interactions of viruses with dendritic cells: a double-edged sword. J Exp Med 186:795–796

Kaiserlian D, Dubois B (2001) Dendritic cells and viral immunity: friends or foes. Semin Immunol 13:303–310

Pulendran B, Palucka K, Banchereau J (2001) Sensing pathogens and tuning immune responses. Science 293:253–256

Schneider-Schaules S, Meulen VT (2002) Triggering of an interference with immune activation: interactions of measles virus with monocytes and dendritic cells. Viral Immunol 15:417–428

Sewel AK, Price DA (2001) Dendritic cells and transmission of HIV-1. Trends Immunol 22: 173–175

Yewdell JW, Hill AB (2002) Viral interference with antigen presentation. Nat Immunol 3: 1019–1025

4. Dendritic Cells and Allergy

The Immune Response During Allergic Manifestations

Through the evolutionary process, two distinct and highly sophisticated defense mechanisms have developed in human beings for survival in hostile environments. One is the innate immune system, which reacts rapidly (from within minutes to a few hours) and in a rather simple way attacks pathogens. The other, the acquired immune system, has evolved to provide a more adaptive and highly specific defense response to agents, antigens (Ags), and other substances that are nonself and dangerous to the host. This adaptive immune system also possesses the unique ability to induce tolerance to self-structures and possibly to nondangerous stimuli. It is important to understand how this balance between immune response and immune tolerance is regulated in vivo. In order to maintain homeostasis in the body, cells of the effector and regulatory limbs of the immune system interact in a coordinated way so that the magnitude and nature of the effector immune response is purposeful and functional in the context of a particular stimulus.

However, some susceptible individuals respond in an inappropriate manner to certain environmental antigens generally known as allergens. Development of allergic manifestations following exposure to allergens is dependent on the personal characteristics of the affected individuals, including their genetic background. Allergic diseases are increasing in prevalence and are now a major source of disability throughout the developed world. Information from the developing world is lacking owing to the poorly developed health care delivery system there. Among allergic diseases, atopic (a term usually used interchangeably with allergic) asthma in the lung and atopic dermatitis (allergic eczema) in the skin are the most serious and prevalent allergic diseases in most countries of the world. In Japan, perennial and seasonal rhinitis in the upper airways and allergic conjunctivitis in the eye are major public health problems. In general, allergic diseases show moderate to severe clinical manifestations, but in their most acute form and in some individuals, they manifest as the life-threatening systemic response called anaphylaxis.

Allergic responses are characteristically triggered by immunoglobulin E (IgE). Susceptible individuals show a genetic tendency to develop elevated levels of allergen-specific IgE. In individuals previously sensitized to an allergen, allergen-specific IgE antibodies bind to high-affinity IgE receptors on the surfaces of mast cells in target tissues and induce the following responses:

1. Deregulation and release of mediators such as histamine, tryptase, and prostaglandins
2. Induction of increased vascular permeability, local edema, and itching

This acute type-1 immediate hypersensitivity response is frequently followed by a late phase reaction, which declines with time. During the late phase response, eosinophil and CD4$^+$ T lymphocytes infiltrate to the site of allergic response. It is important to note that even in the absence of IgE sensitization and an early phase response, allergen-specific T cells may elicit a direct late phase response. Thus, T lymphocyte-mediated immune responses play a key role during the delayed type-IV cell-mediated allergic hypersensitive response.

Data are accumulating regarding the role of tissue microenvironments in allergic manifestations. Even in the absence of a recent allergen provocation, there is an underlying persistent chronic inflammation of the target organs in allergic diseases. These manifestations are mainly due to eosinophils and CD4$^+$ T lymphocytes. Activated eosinophils probably contribute to disease chronicity by damaging epithelial cells and epidermal barriers, thus making the target organ more vulnerable to environmental antigens. In fact, CD4$^+$ T lymphocytes are now regarded as the orchestrator of the chronic allergic immune response. Allergen-specific CD4$^+$ T lymphocytes are able to maintain chronic inflammation in allergic individuals even in the absence of fresh allergen. Allergen-specific T lymphocytes have been cloned from allergic lesions, and these T lymphocytes have been found to be skewed to the Th2 phenotypes. In human, Th2 lymphocytes produce cytokines such as interleukin (IL)-4, IL-5, and IL-13, and these cytokines are responsible for much of the pathophysiology of allergic diseases. Among these, IL-4 is most important in the context of allergic diseases. This cytokine has the following properties relevant to immunopathology of allergy:

1. IL-4 and IL-13 can bind to the α chain of the IL-4 receptor and hence share many biological functions.
2. Not only is IL-4 produced by Th2 cells, it can also promote Th2 differentiation.
3. IL-4 is capable of inducing human B cells to switch immunoglobulin isotype production to IgE.
4. IL-4, along with IL-3, acts as a growth factor for mast cells and leads to upregulation of the expression of vascular cell adhesion molecule (VCAM) 1 on endothelial cells.

In summary, allergic manifestations are seen in genetically susceptible individuals in response to allergens. In the initial phase, histamine released from mast cells might be dominant. However, cytokines produced by Th2 lymphocytes may determine the progression of the allergic response. Even in the absence of primary sensitization, lymphocytes can induce the chronic inflammatory changes seen during allergy attacks.

Involvement of Dendritic Cells in Allergy

Introduction

Factors derived from mast cells and eosinophils appear to induce the manifestations of allergic diseases, whereas lymphocytes and the altered mucosal milieu are

Involvement of DCs in allergy

1. Uptake, processing, and transport of allergens by DCs
2. Th2 polarization by DCs after allergens encountered
3. Induction of macrophage inflammatory protein-3α by allergens
   (a chemotactant for immature DCs)
4. Expression of IgE receptor (FCεR1) by human DCs
5. Allergens attached to FCεR1 on DCs are efficiently internalized

A

Th2 polarization by DCs in allergy

1. Low dose of allergens
2. Low affinity of allergens
3. Prolonged exposure of allergens with TCR ligation
4. High IL-4 and prostaglandins in tissue of allergen deposition
5. Low levels of IL-12 in the tissue of localization of allergens

B

Fig. 4.1A,B. The involvement of dendritic cells (*DCs*) in allergy. **A** DCs might participate in the initiation or perpetuation of allergic manifestations by acting as antigen-presenting cells. DCs would recognize, capture, process, and present allergens for the immune response. In addition, DCs might participate in chronic allergic manifestations by inducing T helper (*Th*) 2 polarization. Some of the allergic manifestations might be mediated by immunoglobulin E (*IgE*) receptors on DCs. **B** Myeloid DCs, which reside at the interface of skin and exposed surface, induce Th1 polarization after engulfing allergens. This might be related to low antigen dose, low affinity of antigen, or prolonged ligation with a T-cell receptor (*TCR*). In addition, allergen-primed DCs may also induce high levels of interleukin (*IL*)-4 and low levels of IL-12

dominant during the progression of acute and chronic allergic diseases. In fact, cytokines and mediators produced by T helper lymphocytes cause the long-lasting inflammation and tissue damage in chronic allergic diseases. As shown in Fig. 4.1, antigen-presenting dendritic cells (DCs) might influence the course of allergic diseases by various mechanisms in vivo. Studies on the induction, maintenance, and regulation of Ag-specific immune responses indicate that DCs are the inducers and regulators of various types of immune responses. The origin, phenotypes, and functions of DCs are described in other chapters of this book; here we provide a short account of DCs that may be helpful for understanding the role of DCs in allergy. Sites affected by allergic diseases typically lie at the interface between the body and the external environment. Huge numbers of DCs are available at these sites. DCs are equipped with an elegant antigen-recognition apparatus comprising pathogen-recognition receptors, which can recognize microbes, transformed cells (apoptotic or tumor-like cells), and Ags. Apart from receptor-mediated recognition of microbial agents, Ags, or transformed cells, DCs sense alterations of the mucosal milieu. After recognizing Ags, transformed cells, or abnormal entities, DCs capture and internalize these agents by using highly specialized mechanisms such as macropinocytosis, receptor-mediated endocytosis, and phagocytosis. Allergens are also internalized by DCs.

The first time a specific allergen is internalized, the DCs determine whether it is a self/nondangerous or nonself/harmful agent for the host. The local tissue microenvironment provides the requisite signals for this determination to the DCs. Based on this determination, the allergen might elicit a tolerance response, or an immune response may be induced. To induce an allergen-specific immune response, DCs cleave the antigens into antigenic peptides, which are expressed on the surfaces of DCs along with the self-major histocompatibility complex (MHC) molecules. DCs expressing the antigenic epitopes of the allergen along with the self-MHC molecules migrate to secondary lymphoid tissues for the induction of the allergen-specific immune response. Experimental evidence supports this scenario for the presentation of allergens in allergic diseases. In the skin, Langerhans cells (LC) have been shown to take up, process, and transport allergens to the local draining lymph nodes, where they present the allergens to naive T cells, indicating a dominant role of DCs in the primary allergen-specific immune response. It is also possible that allergen-specific helper T cells induce the formation of allergen-specific B cells in the immunological synapse in the lymphoid tissues. However, direct proof of these cellular events in vivo is still lacking.

In successive steps, the progeny of naive cells enter the circulation and then the peripheral tissues. The mobilization of allergen-specific $CD4^+$ T lymphocytes and B cells is under the control of sets of adhesion molecules and chemotactic gradients. In the tissues, these cells may immediately perform their effector functions or they may become memory cells. Successive presentation of allergens by DCs leads to the production of various cytokines by T cells, IgE production by B cells, and recruitment of eosinophils and additional memory cells from circulation or from lymphoid tissues. This repeated presentation of allergens by DCs leads to the perpetuation of the allergic manifestations. It is uncertain if DCs are essential for activating allergen-specific memory T cells or if other antigen-presenting cells (APCs) perform this action; B cells are regarded as APCs, but these cells are very rare at sites affected by allergy. Although epithelial cells can express MHC class II molecules, they do not show CD40 or molecules involved in T-cell activation. Macrophages are also unable to induce and maintain a sustained T-cell response. Experimental evidence has shown that alveolar and interstitial macrophages fail to support T-cell proliferation in an antigen-specific manner, although they can support cytokine production. In contrast, macrophages may downregulate the allergic manifestation by producing nitric oxide (NO), because NO can inhibit many DC functions. Some macrophages such as pulmonary macrophages suppress T-cell function. Thus, it appears that antigen presentation by DCs is essential for the stimulation of allergen-specific lymphocytes and for the maintenance of chronic allergic conditions. Experimental evidence supports this assertion because depletion of DCs from antigen-sensitized mice led to a failure to develop eosinophilic infiltration after rechallenge with the original antigen.

However, in humans, it is difficult to prove the involvement of DCs in allergy, especially in secondary allergic inflammation. Because of ethical concerns, these types of studies cannot be conducted in humans. However, experimental evidence supports a role for DCs in human allergy. $CD1a^+$ DCs isolated from bronchoalveolar lavages activate Ag-specific T helper (Th) 2 lymphocytes. Involvement of DCs in the maintenance of the allergic manifestation is predictable from the presence of DCs within epithelial linings, and this positioning of DCs favors their interaction with allergens. Intraepithelial DCs are highly sensitive to the action of inflammatory stimuli. Allergens and other stimuli induce expression of macrophage inflammatory protein (MIP)-3α and might aid to the mobilization of DCs.

DCs and the Regulation of IgE Synthesis

The most notable relationship between DCs and human allergic manifestations is shown by the expression of an IgE receptor (FcεR1) on human DCs. This receptor may play a dominant role in the perpetuation of atopic dermatitis and other allergic manifestations. FcεR1, which is a member of the antigen-receptor superfamily, is a tetrameric complex comprising α and β chains and two disulfide-linked γ chains. In rodents, FcεR1 is confined to the surfaces of mast cells. However, in humans, the mRNA of α and γ subunits of FcεR1 are detected in LCs and circulating DCs. As mentioned above, uptake, processing, and presentation of Ags are the main functions of DCs. DCs utilize nonspecific adsorption, fluid-phase pinocytosis, and cell-surface receptor endocytosis for capturing Ags. Of these, cell surface receptor-mediated endocytosis is the most efficient and specific pathway. The expression of FcεR1 would allow DCs to react with allergens by binding large amounts of IgE molecules with various specificities. This would markedly enhance the probability of cross-linking FcεRI by a defined allergen at the cell surface. The IgE-FcεRI complexes would allow the capture of large allergens, which, under normal circumstances, are not engulfed via the usual pathway, that is, by pinocytosis. Finally, the aggregation of FcεRI on DCs is followed by its internalization via receptor-mediated endocytosis via coated pits, coated vesicles, and endosomes. FcεRI-expressing DCs armed with specific IgE might boost the secondary immune response and trigger further IgE synthesis by recruiting and activating more antigen-specific Th2 cells. Although experimental evidence is lacking, simultaneous antigen uptake and FcεRI aggregation on DCs might lead to the de novo synthesis and release of mediators capable of directing T cells toward a defined phenotype or function, that is, Th1 or Th2 cells.

Th2 Polarization by DCs in the Context of Allergy

DCs initiate the primary immune response and regulate the magnitude of the secondary immune response. When necessary, DCs induce immunological tolerance. Another major function of DCs is to define the nature of the immune response; DCs are vital for the polarization of T cells to Th1 or Th2 cell types. Several factors, such as the nature of the DCs, the microenvironment of the mucosa, the antigen dose, the duration of T-cell receptor (TCR) ligation, and the nature of cytokines in the peripheral and lymphoid tissues, determine the polarization of T cells. In allergic diseases, allergen-specific T cells are polarized toward the Th2 phenotype. More importantly, cytokines produced by Th2 lymphocytes induce and perpetuate the pathological process in allergic diseases. It is possible that DCs induce allergen-specific primary and secondary immune responses through their potent APC capacity.

Plasmacytoid DCs are defined by their negativity with respect to lineage markers and CD11c and by their expression of CD4 and CD123. Plasmacytoid DCs, or DC2 precursors, induce T lymphocytes to differentiate into the Th2 phenotype if treated in vitro with CD40L and IL-3. However, they are able to polarize T cells to the Th1 phenotype if treated with virus. Do plasmacytoid DCs preferentially capture allergens in allergic diseases? IL-3, which is derived from mast cells, induces the maturation of plasmacytoid DCs. As mast cells are detected near allergic tissues, IL-3 derived from those mast cells might cause maturation of plasmacytoid DCs and polarization of T cells to the Th2 phenotype in allergic conditions. However, most allergens are concentrated at the body's epithelial surfaces. DCs at these locations are myeloid, irrespective of their precursors. LCs, which are associated with the pathological processes of allergic dermatitis, are also of myeloid origin. Thus, it appears that myeloid DCs induce Th2 polarization in allergic conditions; however, further understanding of the role of plasmacytoid DCs in allergy is needed.

Th2 Polarization by Myeloid DCs in Allergic Conditions

As DCs in the vicinity of the point of entry of allergens are myeloid DCs, it is important to show how myeloid DCs could induce Th2 polarization after encountering allergens. Antigen presentation by DCs induces Th2 phenotypes under the following conditions:

1. Low Ag dose: The dose of environmental allergens is usually low, and thus it is logical to assume that a low allergen dose might induce allergic lesions. However, this is not true of food allergens because the dose of such antigens is usually very high.

2. Low Ag affinity: Low Ag affinity induces Th2 polarization, but very little information is available regarding comparative affinity levels of allergens and other antigens that induce Th1 and Th2 types of immune responses.

3. Prolonged TCR engagement: Low doses of Ag with low affinity may favor a prolonged TCR engagement, which in turn may cause Th2 polarization. However, this possibility needs to be verified for allergens.

4. Presence of certain soluble factors: IL-4 is the main mediator of the Th2 response in humans. During primary allergic sensitization, natural killer (NK) cells might be a source of IL-4. In established allergic inflammations, mast cells, eosinophils, and Th2 cells can produce IL-4. IL-4 in the tissue microenvironment might cause DCs to induce Th2 polarization. Among DC-derived cytokines, IL-6 may induce Th2 differentiation. In addition, IL-10, by producing IL-4, may also potentiate Th2 polarization. Moreover, DC-derived chemokines such as the monocyte chemotactic protein-1 induce Th2 polarization in vitro.

IL-12 is another important cytokine that mediates the polarization of T cells. Initially, it was assumed that IL-12 induces Th1 polarization, but now experimental evidence has shown that the amount of IL-12 in the tissue microenvironment determines the nature of Th polarization. In allergic diseases, prostaglandins and IL-10 would downregulate the production of IL-12 and might favor Th2 polarization. In addition, histamine, type-1 IFN, and monocyte chemotactic factors 1 to 4 may also promote Th2 polarization.

Dendritic Cells in Animal Models of Allergy

Some insights into the role of DCs in allergic manifestations have been gained from studies of rodent models of allergy. When rodents inhaled ovalbumin, the eosinophilic airway became inflamed. In this animal model, DCs were recruited at the sites of inflammation, and these DCs captured the inhaled ovalbumin. Furthermore, the oval-bumin was processed into an immunogenic form on MHC class II molecules. The role of macrophages in the establishment of inflammation was not clear in this model. However, macrophages produce NO, which blocks the maturation of DCs. Thus, a group of immature DCs in antigen-capturing mode persisted in the tissues for a pro-longed period. These DCs were myeloid, but owing to their immature phenotype, they could not produce IL-12. The lack of IL-12 production by these DCs might have led to the induction of Th2 polarization. The preferential capacity of these DCs to induce a Th2 immune response was further shown by intravenous administration of these DCs, which caused Th2-dependent immunoglobulin production in naive rats.

Administration of ovalbumin-pulsed bone marrow-derived DCs into the trachea resulted in eosinophilic airway inflammation and goblet-cell hyperplasia, which in mice and rats is mediated by Th2 lymphocytes capable of producing IL-4 and IL-5. The sensitization process occurred after migration of the immature DCs into the draining mediastinal lymph nodes.

If we critically analyze these cellular events, some important information about the immune response in allergic conditions is revealed. In general, primary exposure to ovalbumin via the respiratory route is a tolerogenic event. This is especially true if the ovalbumin is allowed to be presented by immature DCs. However, when endoge-nous airway DCs were activated by transgenic expression of granulocyte-macrophage colony-stimulating factor (GM-CSF) or by simultaneous infection with influenza virus, tolerance was circumvented and eosinophilic airway inflammation ensured. From these models, it appears that DCs are responsible for sensitization to inhaled allergens. More importantly, DCs are also attracted from the bone marrow and the bloodstream into sites of eosinophilic airway inflammation during the secondary immune response to ovalbumin. Moreover, DCs ensure the maintenance of eosinophilic airway inflammation and IgE synthesis in sensitized mice. However, the ability of airway DCs to induce polarization toward a Th2 phenotype after intake of the allergen needs to be further explored experimentally.

Dendritic Cells in Human Allergy

Events similar to those shown by several studies of allergic diseases in animal models may also happen in humans. Human DCs might also be implicated in Th2 sensitiza-tion to common allergens in genetically predisposed individuals. To trace the basic mechanism of primary sensitization, we need to look at immunological events during the neonatal period and early infancy, when DCs are functionally immature, making this life stage the peak period of sensitization to allergens. These DCs might fail to counterbalance the default Th0/Th2 priming to common allergens received from the mother or the environment. The increased occurrence of allergic diseases in Western countries might be explained by their relative socioeconomic status, which favors exposure to low doses of allergens. Such low doses might make DCs incapable of pro-ducing adequate IL-12, so they would induce polarization to the Th2 type of immune response. Moreover, prolonged TCR ligation, which may be a common event in cases of low allergen doses, is thought to favor Th2 polarization. Although these events are not well supported by human studies, at least one study supports this scenario. Induction of novel Th2-dependent sensitization to bovine serum albumin was seen after repeated DC injections when bovine serum albumin was used in autologous DC preparations. This led to the production of anti-bovine albumin IgE and anaphylactic reactions in humans.

Allergic Asthma

Most asthmatic patients are atopic, but only some atopic individuals develop allergic asthma. Patients with asthma suffer both acute and chronic phases of this disease, but the pathological lesions differ between the two phases. In the acute phase, histamine is released from the airway mast cells. In the chronic phase, inflammatory infiltrates in the airway mucosa and the altered mucosal milieu influence the pathological process, leading ultimately to permanent injury to the airway mucosa. In asthma, both elevated IgE and a Th2-type immune response are typical. It has already been noted that the high rate of asthma in Western populations might be related to their higher hygienic standards compared with other parts of the world. Low amounts of allergens and the presence of fewer pathogens in the environment may predispose the immune system to a Th2 response. However, genetic factors might also play a role in this regard, especially with respect to the nature of DC maturation in these populations.

However, all these speculations are based on the concept of presentation of allergens by myeloid DCs, which are the main DCs on airway surfaces. With the recent discovery of plasmacytoid DCs, this picture might be altered. Plasmacytoid DCs have now been recognized as a precursor population of DCs that are lineage$^-$, CD11c$^-$ and CD4$^+$, CD123$^+$, HLA DR$^+$. These cells, although they are able to induce both Th1 and Th2 polarization, in most cases induce Th2 polarization. It is still difficult to detect these cells in human tissue sections. Localization of plasmacytoid DCs in bronchial mucosa may provide important insights into the role of plasmacytoid DCs in allergy.

The next important question is how allergens gain access to the airway epithelium. There may be increased transepithelial permeability in asthma. Furthermore, the bronchial epithelium becomes increasingly permeable to macromolecules after allergen deposition. In addition, allergen exposure induces asthmatic epithelial cells to express GM-CSF, which attracts DCs to the site of antigen contact. Studies have now shown that putative MHC class II molecule-bearing DC precursors accumulate in the airway epithelium after exposure to allergens, reaching a maximum within 1 h of Ag exposure. After encountering allergens, DCs change their shape and active DC surveillance within the epithelium is amplified, which results in an increase in the traffic of these cells from the epithelium to the lymph nodes. Rechallenge with the allergens would lead to the recruitment of new DCs from monocytes or other blood precursors, thus amplifying the asthmatic attack. These monocyte-derived DCs from allergic asthma patients show phenotypic differences in the expression of HLA-DR, CD 11b, and the high-affinity receptor for IgE, and even an upregulation of CD86, and they develop into more potent accessory cells than those from normal subjects. Whereas airway DCs are critical in priming the immune system to inhaled allergens, other APC subsets may play a crucial role in the secondary immune response to "known" allergens and thus contribute to the chronicity of asthma.

Atopic Dermatitis

From a pathophysiologic point of view, FcεRI-expressing DCs, and particularly LCs and related DCs in the epidermis, may be dominant players in atopic dermatitis (AD). This possibility is strongly supported by the observation that FcεRI-expressing LCs bearing IgE molecules must be present for eczematous lesions to be provoked by the application of aeroallergens to the skin of AD patients. However, in contrast to other allergic lesions where Th2 polarization is thought to be related to their pathogenesis, both CD4+ and CD8+ T cells play a role in the pathogenesis of AD. Increased numbers of LCs have been reported in the skin of AD patients. A population of CD1a+ dendritic epidermal cells distinct from LCs has also been reported in AD patients. LCs in the skin of AD patients possess an abnormal phenotype and an increased capacity to capture Ags/allergens because of their expression of receptors for specific IgE on their cell surfaces. FcεR1, a high-affinity IgE receptor, and FcεR2, a low affinity IgE receptor, are both upregulated on LCs in AD patients. In addition, CD1a+ LCs express large amounts of costimulatory molecules such as CD86. This capacity of LCs to capture antigens with IgE receptors allows them to drive the activation of T cells. However, it is not clear why LCs favor Th2 polarization, since they produce IL-12. Peripheral blood DCs from AD patients produce high levels of IL-10 and prostaglandin E2, which may favor Th2 polarization. AD is common in children and becomes less severe with age. Abnormal maturation of the immune system during childhood may also underlie the development of AD. In addition to DCs, products of other cells in the skin, such as epithelial cells, fibroblasts, and macrophages, as well as the tissue microenvironment, might also may play a role in the pathogenesis of AD.

Allergic Rhinitis

The role and function of APCs in allergic respiratory diseases is still unclear. Relatively high numbers of both CD1a+ and HLA-DR-expressing DCs have been found in the columnar respiratory epithelium and the lamina propria of the nasal mucosa of patients suffering from grass-pollen allergy. Some DCs of the respiratory epithelium contain Birbeck granules, a feature that classifies them as LCs. Whether the latter represent LCs at a different maturation stage or DCs of a different origin remains to be clarified. The number of airway DCs is highest in the upper airways (600 ± 800 per mm²) and decreases rapidly further down the respiratory tree, suggesting that higher numbers are necessary in the upper airways to cope with the higher Ag exposure there. Indeed, allergen provocation testing in patients has shown that the number of DCs increases after Ag exposure. At the beginning of the provocation period, CD1a+ DCs were observed in the subepithelial layer and around vessels. During the second week of provocation, these cells were found throughout the whole thickness of the epithelium. As there is little evidence that DCs are able to proliferate within the airway mucosa, these changes likely reflect alterations in their recruitment. The pivotal role of airway DCs in antigen processing was further demonstrated by their rapid steady-state turnover rate with a half-life of only 2 days. This contrasts strongly with the situation encountered in keratinized epithelia such as normal human skin, where the corresponding DC populations, for example, LCs, have a half-life of 15 days or longer. The interaction of nasal DCs with other cell types such as mast cells possibly located in the nasal mucosa remains to be elucidated.

There are other allergic conditions in which the roles of DCs have not been explored. Drug-induced allergy, in which patients exhibit allergic manifestations after drug intake, is one such condition. The drugs or their metabolites might be handled by DCs, but the cellular and molecular events regarding these have not been studied. One possibility is that drug metabolites alter the mucosal milieu and thus allow DCs to play a role in the induction of allergic manifestations.

Dendritic Cells as Targets of or Vectors for New Therapeutic Strategies

As a natural adjuvant, DCs play a crucial role in the immunologic surveillance of various tissues, especially those in direct contact with the environment. The roles of DCs in the pathogenesis of allergic contact eczema, as well as of other allergic diseases, are now well documented. Accordingly, these cells could be used as a tool to silence unwanted immunologic reactions.

There are two possible approaches to DC-based therapy for allergic conditions: (1) use of therapeutic agents targeting DC function in vivo and (2) use of DCs that alter the immune status of allergic patients in vivo.

In view of their localization at interface tissues such as the skin and the nasal and lung mucosa, it is comparatively easy to target DCs for therapy. In the skin, ultraviolet radiation is known to alter profoundly the biology of LCs and DCs (as well as that of the surrounding epithelial cells) and is routinely used in the treatment of chronic inflammatory skin diseases. Similarly, glucocorticoids strongly affect the capacity of DCs to induce an immune response, although the exact mechanisms are far from clear. Indeed, DCs exposed to glucocorticoids seem to increase their expression of several functionally relevant molecules such as HLA-DR or CD86, but their stimulatory activity is clearly suppressed. More recently, it has been shown that a new generation of immunosuppressive macrolides, that is, tacrolimus and ascomycin, which in contrast to cyclosporin A, can be used topically, suppress the expression of costimulatory molecules, inhibit the appearance of distinct DCs in inflammatory tissue reactions, and decrease the stimulatory activity of DCs in vitro, as well as in vivo, after local application. Finally, local application of molecules interfering with the binding of IgE to its receptor or compounds inhibiting defined activation mechanisms initiated by FcεRI-expressing DCs in situ could represent valuable alternatives in the future management of atopic conditions.

In addition to various agents that affect DC function, DCs by themselves have the potential to be used as therapeutic agents. Recent progress in understanding the ontogeny of DCs and techniques developed for their generation in vitro have led to an immunologic revolution and opened up new therapeutic options. Such in vitro generated DCs might be used to silence hypersensitivity reactions. A number of pathologic conditions are known to be induced by distinct forms of hypersensitivity reactions. Among them, organ transplantation, autoimmune diseases, and allergic diseases are the most representative examples. DCs with appropriate phenotypic and functional modulation by cytokines such as IL-10 or transforming growth factor-β may be suitable for silencing auto- and alloreactive, as well as allergen-specific, T cells.

Recommended Readings

Lambrecht BN (2001) The dendritic cells in allergic airway diseases: a new player to the game. Clin Exp Allergy 31:206–218

Lambrecht BN (2001) Allergen uptake by dendritic cells. Curr Opin Allergy Clin Immunol 1:51–59

Novak N, Haberstok J, Geiger E, et al. (1999) Dendritic cells in allergy. Allergy 54:792–803

Semper AE, Gudin AM, Holloway JA, et al. (2001) Dendritic cells in allergy. In: Lotze MT, Thomson AW (eds) Dendritic cells. Academic Press, San Diego, CA, USA, pp 523–528

Wollenberg A, Kraft S, Oppel T, et al. (2000) Atopic dermatitis: pathogenetic mechanisms. Clin Dermatol 25:530–534

5. Dendritic Cells in Autoimmunity

General Considerations

Association of Dendritic Cells with Autoimmunity

Autoimmunity is characterized by the presence of autoreactive B cells and/or auto-reactive T cells and the corresponding organ manifestations. Autoreactive B cells produce autoantibodies, whereas autoreactive T cells may induce cellular damage. Under normal conditions, the immune response is not initiated by antigens such as self-antigens and nondangerous entities. In the steady state, presentation of these antigens would lead to immunogenic tolerance. This situation requires that the host accurately distinguish self from nonself. The host should also discriminate between dangerous and nondangerous entities. Nevertheless, self-antigens have potential immunogenicity and are capable of inducing immune responses and autoimmunity. When immunity is initiated to self-antigens in a host, there might be pathogenic consequences such as autoimmune disease. In other words, autoimmunity is the broken state of immunological unresponsiveness (tolerance) to self-antigens.

Antigen-presenting dendritic cells (DCs) are the critical decision-making cells during both the induction of an immune response and the induction of immunological unresponsiveness or tolerance. Thus, it is natural that when there is the induction of autoimmune processes, DCs would have a dominant role. In the steady state, the primary function of DCs is to induce immune nonresponsiveness to self-antigens and harmless entities. Moreover, DCs regulate both central and peripheral tolerance. Thus, DCs prevent the induction of autoimmune processes under physiological conditions. However, in genetically susceptible hosts, or in response to some alteration of the mucosal milieu, DCs might not be able to distinguish between self and nonself antigens properly. Also, the presence of certain inflammatory mediators in the mucosal milieu might cause DCs to induce an immune response to self-antigens or to harmless entities.

Although DCs participate in the induction or perpetuation of autoimmunity, DCs should also be able to downregulate this process. DCs can be altered in vitro, and possibly in vivo, from immunological to tolerogenic mode. Therefore, DC-based therapy or DC-targeting therapy may aid in the management of some autoimmune diseases, even if DCs did not contribute in any major way to the induction of those auto-immune processes. As autoantigens are diverse with respect to their antigenicity, amounts, and affinity, it is vitally important to investigate DC–autoantigen interactions case by case. More importantly, in most autoimmune diseases, the autoantigens are unknown. Also, several autoantigens may be implicated in one autoimmune disease. Therefore, the role of DCs in the induction or perpetuation of autoimmune processes needs to be explored experimentally.

Outline of DC Research in Autoimmune Diseases

Autoimmune diseases are a growing public health problem, especially as the population ages. Women are more affected by autoimmune diseases than men. Although there are very few reports on the role of hormones in the activation and maturation of DCs, circumstantial evidence suggests such a role, especially for female hormones, in the initiation or perpetuation of autoimmune diseases. It is known that high doses of prolactin lead to the maturation of DCs. Thyroid hormones also induce DCs to produce interleukin (IL)-12, which explains the high serum level of IL-12 in patients with hyperthyroidism. Treatment of DCs with nonsteroidal anti-estrogens, including tamoxifen, inhibits their terminal maturation. Hormones can also downregulate DC activation. Unfortunately, no explanation is available for these observations. Studies on the activation and deactivation of DCs are of minimal importance if the types of DCs used in them are not standardized. Also, it is important to know what DC functions were evaluated. In general, upregulation of surface antigens on DCs or increased allostimulatory capacity of DCs are regarded as signs of DC activation, but these phenomena have very few practical implications in the context of autoimmunity.

Autoimmune diseases show two peaks with respect to age distribution: they occur especially in people in their twenties to thirties and their fifties. Systemic lupus erythematosus (SLE) and HLA DR3[+] autoimmune hepatitis have their peak onset in patients in their twenties, and HLA DR4[+] autoimmune hepatitis and primary biliary cirrhosis (PBC) usually occur in patients in their fifties. In general, DC frequency and functioning are downregulated as people age, but no study has attempted to evaluate whether the functioning of both immunogenic and tolerogenic DCs are downregulated with age. On the other hand, DCs and circulatory T cells have more chances to encounter autoantigens in vivo in aging patients. As people age, more of their cells undergo apoptosis as well. DCs are thus more likely to engulf autoantigens. Many inflammatory diseases also occur more frequently in older people. Such diseases provide an inflammatory mucosal milieu which may cause autoantigens to become immunogenic in vivo.

Changes in the number and functioning of DCs have been studied for several human autoimmune diseases as well as in animal models of autoimmune diseases. There are striking similarities in the behavior of DCs in affected organs among autoimmune diseases, although their pathogenesis differs. DCs accumulate in diseased tissues in autoimmune diseases, especially those with activation and maturation markers (Table 5.1). DCs in affected tissues express MHC class II and costimulatory molecules, including CD80 and CD86. Interestingly, DCs with different phenotypes and diverse levels of activation have been observed in diseased tissues.

The final goal of research on DCs in autoimmunity is to develop therapy for autoimmune diseases. Some therapeutic trials have been carried out, mainly in animal models. Many immunosuppressive drugs, including azathioprine, mizoribine, and

Table 5.1. Dendritic cells (DCs) in autoimmune diseases

Features of DCs	Diseases or disease model	Alterations
DCs in peripheral blood		
Frequency of myeloid DC precursors	Primary biliary cirrhosis	Decreased
Stimulatory capacity of DCs	Primary biliary cirrhosis	Decreased
	Ulcerative colitis	Increased
DCs in diseased organs	Rheumatoid arthritis	[Quantification and
[Localization of DCs]	Crohn's diseases	comparison could
	Ulcerative colitis	not be done]
	Psoriasis	
	Chronic thyroiditis	
	Primary biliary cirrhosis	
	Autoimmune gastritis in mice	
	Type 1 DM in mice	
Plasmacytoid DCs in diseased organs	Cutaneous lupus erythematosus	[Quantification could not be done]
	Primary biliary cirrhosis	
Functioning of DCs from diseased organs	Psoriasis (dermal DCs)	Increased
	Rheumatoid arthritis (synovial DCs)	Increased
Therapy targeting or using DCs		
Depletion of matured DCs from peripheral blood	Human ulcerative colitis	Clinical and histological improvement
Changes in DCs due to drugs [Bezafibrate improves NO production by DCs]	Human primary biliary cirrhosis	Clinical improvement
IFN-γ-stimulated DCs	Mouse diabetic model	Disease suppression
Antigen-loaded immature DCs	Experimental autoimmune uveoretinitis	Disease protection

DM, diabetes mellitus; IFN, interferon; NO, nitric oxide

cyclosporine, affect DC functioning. Glucocorticoids and vitamin D suppress the maturation and differentiation of DCs. However, all these drugs have multiple effects. Indeed, drugs that specifically affect DC functioning have not yet been identified. It may be possible to use tolerogenic DCs as therapeutic agents in autoimmune diseases. However, it is still uncertain whether organ-specific DCs would be required to treat organ-specific autoimmune diseases.

DCs in the Pathogenesis of Autoimmune Diseases

DCs During Initiation and Perpetuation of Autoimmunity

In spite of the defense measures taken by the body to maintain tolerance to self, autoimmunity is an ever-present reality. Various explanations have been proposed to account for the initiation of an autoimmune response: sequestered antigen, molecular mimicry, altered self-antigen, self-antigen with increased MHC class II expression, and decreased suppression of immunity. Loss of tolerance to self-antigens is critical in the pathogenesis of autoimmunity. While autoimmunity may occur through many mechanisms, the key features are that the autoantigen is presented persistently, and the consequences of this presentation are inflammation and tissue damage, for which certain critical cytokines and immune mediators are responsible.

DCs play essential roles in both the initiation and perpetuation of autoimmunity and autoimmune diseases. The mechanisms underlying the breakdown of self-tolerance and the induction of autoimmunity are not well understood, and the exact role of DCs in this process is yet to be clarified. However, several hypotheses suggest the involvement of DCs in autoimmunity, including the self/nonself theory and the danger/nondanger hypothesis. According to the self/nonself theory, the immune response is not initiated to self-antigens, rather nonself antigens induce the immune response. Thus, some of the host's cells should be able to distinguish between self and nonself antigens. DCs act as the sentinels of the immune system, and they are equipped with potent antigen-recognition apparatuses. Naturally, DCs have the primary responsibility for recognizing various antigens in vivo. Several investigations have shown that viral, bacterial, and parasitic antigens are recognized by DCs with pathogen-recognition receptors. On the other hand, pathogenic organisms express the ligands of pathogen-recognition receptors. However, almost nothing is known about the ligands of self-antigens and their relevant receptors on DCs. The important question is whether DCs use similar pathogen-recognition receptors for the recognition of both self-antigens and nonself antigens. As there are different types of DCs, some of which are immunogenic and others that are tolerogenic, self-antigens may be recognized by tolerogenic DCs in the steady state. However, it is also possible that self-antigens may be taken up by any type of DC, but that the subsequent steps of antigen handling are different between self and nonself-antigens.

According to the danger model of immune response, an alteration to the tissue microenvironment by trauma, pathogens, toxins, or inflammatory mediators changes the activation status of tissue-residing DCs. This may cause early infiltration and abnormal accumulation of DCs prior to the migration of macrophages and B and T cells into these areas. The environmental changes may also cause changes in the antigen recognition capacity of the DCs. However, it is important to know whether these environmental changes can change the nature of the self-antigens. Do self-antigens look like nonself antigens because of alterations to the environment?

The early infiltration of differentiated DCs into the synovial tissue prior to the exacerbation of disease has been observed in patients with rheumatoid arthritis. Thus, microenvironments, which induce the migration, accumulation, and maturation of DCs, might be important in the initiation of autoimmunity and the onset of autoimmune diseases. Microenvironmental changes may also be induced by necrosis and apoptosis of host cells and by carcinogenesis. In general, DCs promote the stimulatory responses of CD4$^+$ and CD8$^+$ T cells following exposure to necrotic cells, whereas DCs that have encountered apoptotic cells do not induce such stimulatory responses in lymphocytes. However, extremely high amounts of apoptotic cells might induce maturation of DCs even in the absence of further inflammatory signals.

The thymus may play a dominant role during the initiation of autoimmunity. During T-cell development, thymic DCs participate in the deletion of autoreactive T cells. The large T-cell repertoire that develops daily in the thymus contains a huge proportion of self-reactive T cells. Deletion of autoreactive T cells requires the expression and presentation of the relevant autoantigens in the thymus. Recent data have shown that most tissue-specific antigens can be found at the messenger RNA level in the epithelial cells of the thymic medulla. Bone marrow-derived DCs in the thymus express proteins derived from peripheral tissue. It thus appears that thymic DCs delete self-reactive T cells. However, central tolerance is still incompletely understood. Thymic negative selection cannot lead to the deletion of T cells only if the antigen is presented in insufficient amounts by thymic DCs. When central tolerance fails, autoimmunity or autoimmune diseases might result.

It is possible that immature DCs constantly circulate through the tissues of the body and load themselves with self-antigens and other harmless environmental substances. When they encounter T cells, the DCs would deliver signals that might result in the those T cells being deleted or becoming anergic. This ability has been established most clearly for the so-called myeloid DCs. However, it is unknown whether DCs derived from monocytes ever have a phase during which they are able to tolerize T cells. Indeed, the antigens that are delivered to T cells originate at the site of activation. The fact that DC maturation signals in affected tissue induce autoimmunity to autoantigens reflects the widespread availability of autoantigens throughout the body. Ingestion of apoptotic bodies is a feature of DCs. These apoptotic bodies contain bulk amounts of autoantigens. Although DCs ingesting apoptotic bodies should induce tolerance to the ingested antigens in steady state, if inflammatory stimuli are present in the tissue of ingestion of apoptotic bodies, this situation could change. Thus, DCs that have ingested apoptotic cells may induce autoantibodies and accelerate autoimmunity in vivo.

Although mature DCs do not seem to be affected by IL-10, a Th2-promoting cytokine, this cytokine can cause fewer DCs to mature during the initial stages of DC activation. This suggests their role in the induction of immune tolerance. The repeated stimulation of T cells by immature DCs results in the generation of regulatory IL-10-producing CD4$^+$, CD25$^+$ T cells, which can promote tolerogenicity. There are two main theories as to how peripheral regulation of immune responses occurs. First, since DCs containing apoptotic bodies constitutively migrate from peripheral sites to draining lymph nodes, and since processed self-antigens derived from somatic cells are constitutively cross-presented, mechanisms must be in place to prevent cross-priming to somatic self-antigens in lymphoid organs. RelB activity is required for myeloid DC differentiation. Constitutive presentation of self-antigens may occur by putative immature or regulatory nuclear RelB-DCs draining from the periphery to draining lymph nodes. RelB-DCs thus help maintain peripheral tolerance. Second, following induction of an effector response, mechanisms must be in place to prevent ongoing induction of an antigen-specific effector response and to limit pathogenic anti-self immune responses at inflammatory sites. Maintaining peripheral tolerance to avoid exaggerated anti-self responses involves a number of distinct mechanisms: immunological ignorance (insufficient numbers of autoantigens in secondary lymphoid organs), the induction of T-cell unresponsiveness (anergy), and dominant T helper (Th) 2-type cytokines. Numerous publications have demonstrated the importance of CD4$^+$, CD25$^+$ regulatory T cells in controlling immune homeostasis and preventing autoimmune diseases. DCs, in their role as controllers of regulatory T cells, might directly or indirectly be players in the initiation and perpetuation of autoimmunity and autoimmune diseases.

DCs in the Tissues in the Early Phase of Autoimmunity

Although DCs with different levels of maturation and activation have been detected in the peripheral blood and in the tissues of patients with autoimmune diseases, these may simply reflect the altered functioning of DCs from the sustained presence of autoimmune disease. Thus, characterizing DCs in patients with autoimmune diseases would provide very little information on the role of DCs in the initiation of such diseases. Accordingly, several investigators have tried to study early cellular events in animal models of autoimmune diseases.

Neonatal Balb/c mice, thymectomized on day 3 after birth, develop progressive autoimmune gastritis. The lesion is characterized by infiltration of mononuclear cells into the gastric tissues. CD11c$^+$ DCs have been localized in this mouse as early as 3 weeks after thymectomy, and their numbers increase with time (Fig. 5.1). The DCs are usually distributed perivascularly, and they are often clustered with CD4$^+$ T cells. It is still unknown whether these DCs migrate from some other sources to the stomach, or whether DC progenitors or precursors in stomach tissue become CD11c$^+$ DCs after the thymectomy. In general, CD11c$^+$ DCs are almost invisible in the normal gastric mucosa. The mobilization of DCs to the tissues might be an important step in the initiation of immune-mediated inflammation of that organ. The observation of chemokine expression in diseased organs and of chemokine receptors on DCs would be important for understanding how early migration of DCs might occur under these conditions. DCs in the stomach tissue of thymectomized Balb/c mice may induce adaptive immunity by capturing, processing, and presenting autoantigens. However, DCs also produce several chemokines that may attract T lymphocytes and allow the localization of macrophages by inhibiting their random migration. Accordingly, early mobilization of DCs may induce tissue damage in the autoimmune condition in various ways.

DCs in Diseased Tissues of Patients with Autoimmune Diseases

DCs, activated DCs, and matured DCs have been localized in the tissues of animal models of autoimmune diseases and in the tissues of human patients with autoimmune diseases. CD11c$^+$ DCs were found to be localized in the portal areas in senescent female C57BL/6 mice, which spontaneously develop PBC-like liver disease. DCs were frequently observed close to the bile duct epithelia (Fig. 5.2). Among these DCs, some showed matured and activated phenotypes, indicated by the expression of MHC class II, CD80, and CD86 molecules. Electron microscope studies showed that these DCs were in contact with lymphocytes (Fig. 5.2). However, the DC functions in the liver tissues of these mice have not been evaluated.

Although DCs enriched from peripheral blood of PBC patients had impaired allostimulatory function, CD11c$^+$ DCs in liver from an animal model of PBC had an activated phenotype. This may indicate that the phenotype and function of blood-derived DCs and tissue DCs might be different under pathological conditions.

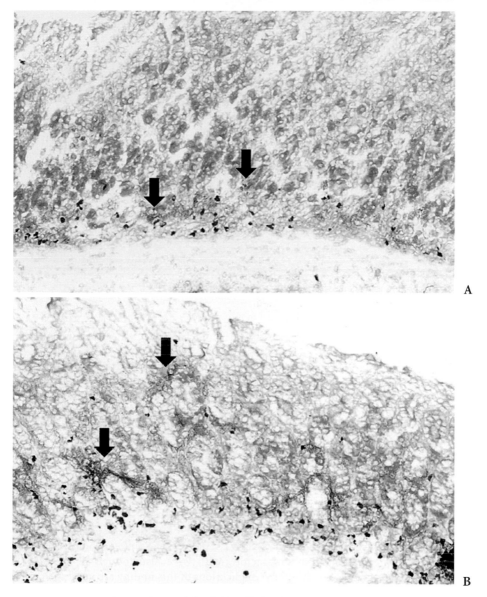

A

B

Fig. 5.1A–C. Accumulation of CD11c⁺ dendritic cells (DCs) in the gastric mucosa in Balb/c mice after neonatal thymectomy in an animal model of autoimmune gastritis. CD11c⁺ DCs were detected by immunostaining using monoclonal antibody. Signals are shown by bluish stainings. CD11c⁺ DCs were detected as early as 4 weeks after thymectomy (**A**). The number of CD11c⁺ DCs were increased at 8 weeks (**B**) and 12 weeks (**C**) after thymectomy. *Arrows*, CD11c⁺ DC. Original magnification ×110

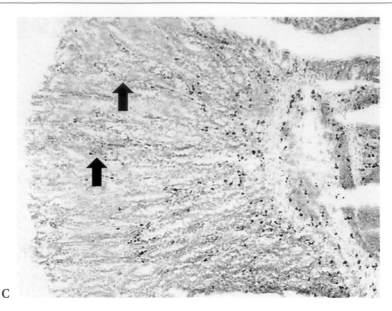

C

Fig. 5.1A–C. *Continued*

However, a question always persists regarding the utility of these animal models. In fact, the development of appropriate animal models of autoimmune diseases would provide more insights into the role of DCs in autoimmunity.

On the other hand, DCs may be different during the initiation of the autoimmune disease (animal model of PBC) compared with after the autoimmune disease has become established (patients with PBC). In conformity with data from the animal model of PBC, mature DCs expressing CD83 have also been found in liver tissues of patients with PBC (Fig. 5.3A). It has also been reported that CD86$^+$ DCs may be more relevant in early stages of PBC because they disappear from the liver at later stages. These puzzling issues regarding the phenotypes and functions of DCs in autoimmune diseases should be studied in appropriate animal models.

Mature DCs expressing CD83 have been localized in inflamed colonic mucosa of patients with ulcerative colitis (UC) (Fig. 5.3B). DCs expressing both CD83 and macrophage migration inhibitory factor (MIF) were also located in the colonic mucosa of UC patients. Although the implications of this finding are not known, MIF produced by DCs might help mobilize macrophages at the site of tissue injury in patients with UC. Thus, DCs and macrophages might collaborate in the pathogenesis of this disease. DCs expressing dendritic cell-specific intracellular adhesion molecule (ICAM)-3-grabbing nonintegrin (DC-SIGN), IL-12, and IL-18 are more numerous in the colonic mucosa of patients with Crohn's disease.

CD11c$^+$ DCs coexpressing MHC class II, CD80, and CD86 have been found in the tissues of mouse models with autoimmune gastritis, rheumatoid arthritis, chronic thyroiditis, and type-I diabetes mellitus. Phenotypically, these DCs are activated and matured, but their functional capacities have not been explored.

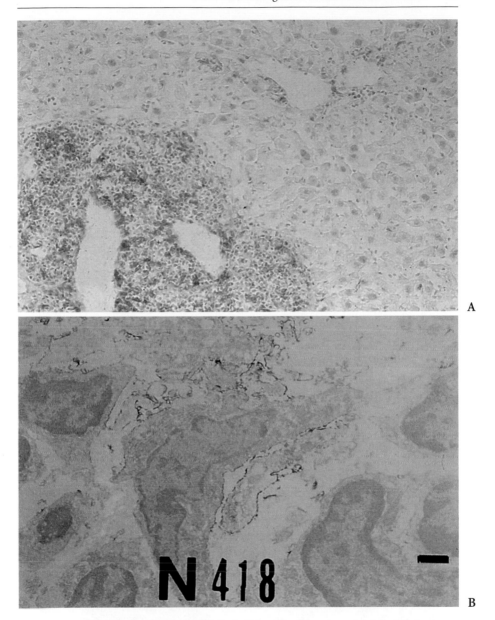

Fig. 5.2A,B. Accumulation of CD11c[+] DCs in the liver tissues from an animal model of primary biliary cirrhosis (PBC), in which PBC-like lesions develop spontaneously in senescent mice C57BL/6 mice. CD11c[+] DCs, shown by brownish stainings, were mainly accumulated near the portal areas (**A**). CD11c[+] DCs (blackish signals) and lymphocytes were in close contact, as shown by immune electron microscopy (**B**). *N418* is the antibody that defect CD11c. Original magnification ×100. *Bar*, 2 µm

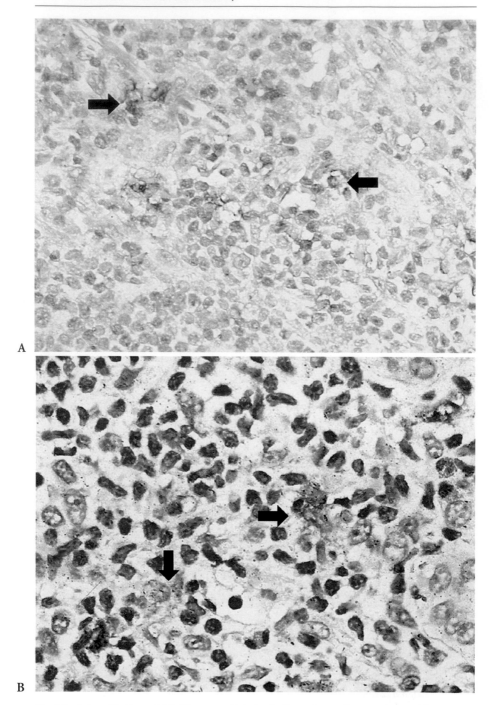

Fig. 5.3. **A** Localization of CD83[+] mature DCs in the liver tissues from patients with PBC and **B** at the colonic mucosa from patients with ulcerative colitis (UC). CD83[+] DCs were localized in the liver tissue in a paraffin-embedded, formalin-fixed specimen by the antigen retrieval technique. Frozen sections of colonic mucosa was used to locate CD83[+] DCs in UC. CD83[+] DCs are shown by *arrows*. Original magnification ×450

In humans, tissue-derived DCs isolated from autoimmune disease patients, including those with rheumatoid synovium and psoriatic dermatitis, have been shown to have a mature phenotype. These DCs have a higher T-cell stimulatory capacity compared with autologous DCs enriched from peripheral blood.

DCs localized in diseased organs might participate in the pathogenesis of autoimmune diseases. However, the clinical implications of this have not been explored. It is true that autoantigens may be most abundant in the injured tissues. These DCs may persistently capture and present autoantigens, thus perpetuating the pathological processes. However, mature DCs might also provide an inflammatory mucosal milieu for the action of activated lymphocytes and macrophages at the tissue level in autoimmune diseases. The importance of DCs in the pathogenesis of autoimmune diseases is further supported by their ability to transfer disease to naive animals. DCs sequester self-peptides responsible for the priming of the specific T-cell responses that lead to autoimmune diseases.

It is now evident that DCs are localized in the diseased tissues of patients with autoimmune diseases. Moreover, both mature and activated DCs have been found in such tissues. However, it is also true that DCs, including mature and activated DCs, are found in diseased tissues of most types of inflammatory diseases, even those with no autoimmune pathology. The quantitative evaluation of the frequencies of mature and activated DCs in tissue is not a simple task because only a very few DC markers are known. Moreover, DCs are highly migratory; thus, the practical implications of mature DCs in the diseased tissues of patients with autoimmune diseases deserve further investigation. More importantly, DCs should not undergo maturation in diseased tissue. Until the dilemma regarding the localization of tissue-located mature DCs is solved, mere localization of mature DCs in the diseased tissue offers very little insight into the role of these DCs in autoimmunity.

Peripheral Blood DCs in Autoimmune Diseases

The frequency and functioning of DCs have been studied in various autoimmune diseases in human. DCs are enriched from precursor populations in the blood, but it is now possible to isolate DC precursors directly from the blood. Precursors of myeloid DCs (lineage , $CD4^+$, $CD11C^+$, HLA DR^+) are less numerous in the peripheral blood of patients with PBC, perhaps owing to their mobilization to the liver tissues. However, this mobilization could not be confirmed because of methodological problems detecting myeloid DCs in the liver.

The functions of DCs enriched by culturing monocytes or an adherent population of peripheral blood mononuclear cells have been evaluated in PBC. The capacity of monocyte-derived DCs to stimulate allogenic T cells was significantly decreased compared with control subjects. Increased production of nitric oxide by DCs from PBC patients was responsible for this decrease (Fig. 5.4). Mature DCs in the liver tissues also expressed inducible nitric oxide (NO) synthase, indicating their capacity to produce NO in the liver tissue (Fig. 5.5). In addition to performing functional studies of peripheral blood DCs, investigators can also use DCs to detect autoantigen-specific T lymphocytes in patients with PBC. Patients with PBC usually have antibodies to pyruvate dehydrogenase complex (PDC) in their sera and PDC-specific T

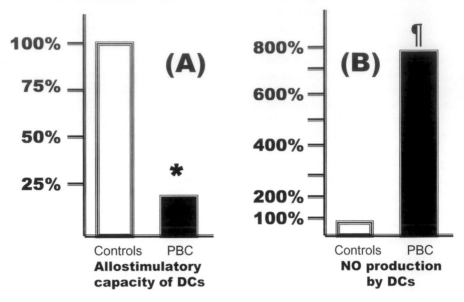

Fig. 5.4A,B. Decreased allostimulatory capacity of DCs in patients with PBC. The mean level of blastogenesis in allogenic MLR containing DCs from controls is shown as 100%. The levels of blastogenesis in cultures containing DCs form PBC patients were calculated based on the allostimulatory capacity of DCs from the controls (**A**). Increased production of nitric oxide (NO) by DCs from PBC patients (**B**). The mean level of NO produced by controls is shown as 100%. *$P < 0.05$; ¶ $P < 0.01$

cells in the liver. However, most patients with PBC do not show a peripheral blood T-cell response to PDC when the conventional lymphoproliferative assays are done with PDC. However, with PDC-pulsed, monocyte-derived DCs, PDC-specific T cells were detected in the peripheral blood of most patients with PBC, even when anti-PDC antibodies could not be detected by conventional methods. This study provides definitive proof of the existence of autoantigen-specific lymphocytes in PBC patients.

In autoimmune hepatitis (AIH) patients, the number and nature of DC precursors was evaluated by flow cytometry. The numbers of myeloid DC and plasmacytoid DC precursors did not differ between patients and controls, but the expression of HLA DR on myeloid DC precursors from patients with AIH, but not on those from patients with PBC, was decreased. However, the expression of HLA DR and CD123 on plasmacytoid DC precursors was significantly decreased in patients with PBC or AIH compared with healthy subjects. As plasmacytoid DCs play a role in the induction of immunogenic tolerance and Th2 polarization, defective expression of surface antigens on plasmacytoid DCs may underlie the switching to the Th1 type of immune response in these autoimmune diseases.

On the other hand, a completely different picture regarding DCs was seen in UC, another autoimmune disease of the colon. When a precursor population of DCs from the peripheral blood of UC patients was cultured to enrich DCs, the number of DCs

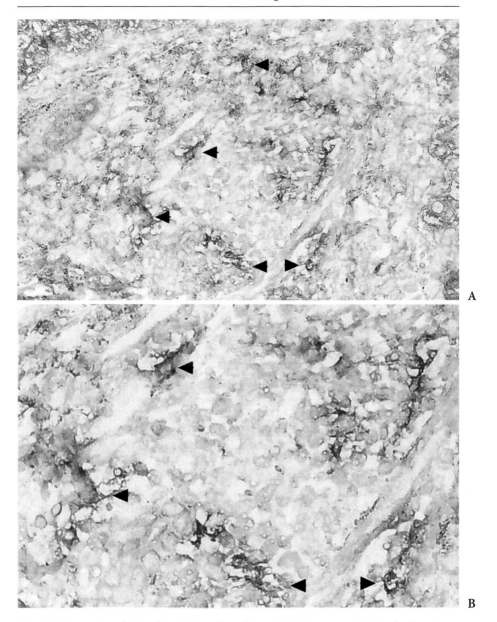

Fig. 5.5. Expression of inducible nitric acid synthase (iNOS) by mature DCs in the liver tissue of patients with PBC. Signals for iNOS and CD83 are shown by bluish and reddish staining, respectively. Some CD83-positive DCs also expressed iNOS. *Arrowheads*, CD11c[+] DC. Original magnification ×450

expressing CD83 antigen was significantly higher than in the controls. The T-cell stimulatory capacity of DCs was thus significantly higher in UC patients compared with controls.

In human autoimmune diseases, understanding of the nature and function of DCs is valuable for patient follow-up, for gaining insight into the progression of these diseases, and for judging the efficacy of therapy. However, this understanding might not lead to greater understanding of the disease mechanism. The number and functional levels of immune cells from the peripheral blood infrequently mirror those from the diseased organ tissues. Thus, it would be much better to evaluate DCs in the affected tissues; however, more DC-specific markers would be required for such studies.

Interferon-α and Plasmacytoid DCs in Autoimmune Diseases

Interferon (IFN)-α is predictably involved in the pathogenesis of autoimmunity, although the prime function of this cytokine is to act during the induction of innate immunity. IFN-α is produced in and around the tissues suffering microbial invasion, and this cytokine can destroy the microbes directly. As microbial infections are thought to influence the induction of autoimmunity, IFN-α may also be involved in this process. Moreover, IFN-α can provide the requisite danger or alarm signals for the induction of adaptive immune responses. It has been long known that type-1 IFN is produced by leukocytes or fibroblasts, but little was known regarding the nature of IFN-producing cells. Only recently it has been become evident that plasmacytoid DCs, which are precursors of circulating DCs, are the most potent producers of IFN-α. Thus, these DCs are also called natural interferon-producing cells. Increased levels of IFN-α have been detected in the sera of patients with SLE. Plasmacytoid DCs produce huge amounts of IFN-α when cultured with sera from SLE patients; possibly the DNA–anti-DNA complexes in SLE sera provide an activation signal for IFN-α production. Moreover, immune complexes in SLE sera may trigger myeloid DCs or other cells to produce IFN-α. Plasmacytoid DCs that produce IFN-α have also been detected in the skin of patients with cutaneous lupus erythematosus.

In addition to SLE, a role for IFN-α in autoimmunity can be postulated from the fact that IFN-α exacerbates or induces acute onset of latent or remission stage autoimmune liver diseases. Plasmacytoid DCs expressing CD123 and CD68 have also recently been found in the liver tissues of patients with PBC.

DC-Targeting and DC-Based Therapy for Autoimmunity

The primary goal in investigating DCs in autoimmune diseases is to understand the pathological processes underlying the diseases and to learn how DCs are involved in those processes. The ultimate goal is to develop therapies for autoimmune diseases that either target or use DCs.

Therapies targeting DCs, although preliminary, have been developed by some investigators. Our research group developed a therapy for nonobese diabetic (NOD) mice that used DCs and one for patients with UC that targeted DCs. The transfer of IFN-γ-stimulated DCs into NOD mice provided long-lasting protection against clinical and histological signs of type-1 diabetes mellitus (DM) in the recipient mice. These findings suggest that the development of autoimmune diabetes in the NOD mouse may controlled in some way by DCs, and the onset of type-1 DM might be controlled by appropriately manipulating DCs in vivo. This approach opens up several options for the therapeutic application of DCs in human type-1 DM. In the experimental autoimmune uveitis mouse model, peptide antigen-bearing immature DCs, but not mature DCs, protect animals from developing uveitis, possibly by inducing high levels of IL-10 and IL-5.

Depletion of leukocytes during lymphocytapheresis is now used as a therapy for UC patients. Interestingly, activated and mature CD83$^+$ DCs are also depleted during this procedure. Lymphocytapheresis is safe and caused clinical, endoscopic, or histologic improvement in all patients studied. This therapy also downregulated the functioning of DCs and decreased levels of IL-6 and IL-8 (Fig. 5.6). Depletion of both activated DCs and lymphocytes may contribute to the therapeutic activity of lymphocytapheresis, but the relative contribution of each still needs to be determined.

Increased production of NO by monocyte-derived DCs was detected in patients with PBC. We speculated that a therapeutic model for PBC could be developed by downregulating NO production from DCs in PBC patients. To achieve this, we used bezafibrate in patients with PBC. This drug causes decreased NO production by DCs and improves the clinical symptoms of PBC patients.

IL-10 is an anti-inflammatory cytokine that is produced by immature liver DC progenitors. Liver DC progenitors also induce IL-10 production by T lymphocytes. We established an autoimmune model of acute hepatitis by injecting C57BL/6 mice with

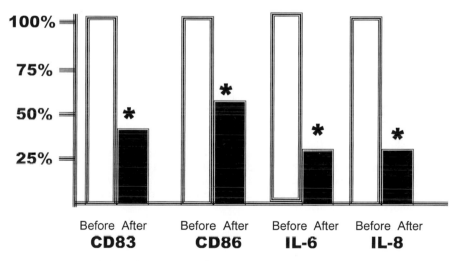

Fig. 5.6. Downregulation of activation and maturation of DCs in patients with UC by lymphocytapheresis. The proportions of CD83$^+$ DCs and CD86$^+$ DCs among total DCs were calculated by flow cytometry before and after lymphocytapheresis. The levels of IL-6 and IL-8 were estimated in the sera. The mean levels of these parameters in UC patients before the start of therapy are shown as 100%. The levels of these parameters after therapy were calculated by comparing them with the levels before therapy. Mature DCs and cytokines decreased significantly after lymphacytapheresis. * $P < 0.05$

concanavalin A (Con-A). Glycyrrhizin, a drug known to improve subjective symptoms of hepatitis, is usually used in patients with hepatitis. Administration of glycyrrhizin, before induction of hepatitis by Con-A prevented hepatitis in C57BL/6 mice. The protective activity of glycyrrhizin was attributed to its capacity to induce IL-10 from liver DCs.

In the future, tolerogenic DCs prepared by manipulating DCs in vitro might be used as a therapeutic tool for autoimmune diseases. Tolerogenic DCs can exploit the same mechanisms that normal DCs employ to induce or maintain tolerance in the steady state, and they would be an invaluable tool for autoimmune disease therapy. Tolerogenic DCs, including immature, IL-10-treated, and TNF-α-treated DCs, may induce peripheral tolerance.

Concluding Remarks

Studies of the immune pathogenesis of various autoimmune diseases have shown that DCs may play a fundamental role in the initiation and perpetuation of autoimmunity and autoimmune diseases. The identification of autoantigens in these pathological conditions would affirm the role of DCs in autoimmune diseases. Recent progress in the molecular biology of the human genome suggests that single nucleotide polymorphisms in sensitive genes contribute to autoimmune diseases. Fusion between immunological and genomic studies may lead to rapid progress in understanding autoimmune diseases. Many DC-based immunotherapy possibilities are available for clinical experiments. The prospect of immunotherapy using antigen-pulsed DCs, tolerogenic DCs, or antigen-specific immunosuppression via DCs is exciting.

Recommended Readings

Kuwana M (2002) Induction of anergic and regulatory T cells by plasmacytoid dendritic cells and other dendritic cell subsets. Hum Immunol 63:1156–1163

Ludewig B, Krebs P, Junt T, et al. (2003) Dendritic cell homeostasis in the regulation of self-reactivity. Curr Pharm Des 9:221–231

Mehling A, Beissert S (2003) Dendritic cells under investigation in autoimmune diseases. Crit Rev Biochem Mol Biol 38:1–21

Thomas R, Lipsky P (1996) Could endogenous self-peptides presented by dendritic cells initiate rheumatoid arthritis? Immunol Today 17:559–564

Thomson AG, Thomas R (2002) Induction of immune tolerance by dendritic cells: implications for preventative and therapeutic immunotherapy of autoimmune disease. Immunol Cell Biol 80:509–519

6. Dendritic Cells in Tumor Immunology

Tumorigenesis and Dendritic Cells

Immunological Events During Tumorigenesis

The mechanisms underlying tumorigenesis of various organs and tissues might share some common features, but it is likely that some organ-specific factors influence tumorigenesis in a particular organ. For example, the cellular and molecular events underlying the development of solid tumors would be different from those underlying tumors of blood cells. Some tumors develop from a malignant state, whereas in other cases, apparent premalignant conditions, even if present, are not well characterized. For example, tumors of liver cells, hepatocellular carcinoma (HCC), usually develop from a definitive precancerous state. Similarly, microbial infections or chemical carcinogens might induce chronic inflammatory changes in several organs that could make them susceptible to malignant transformation. In addition, various other factors, most of which are still elusive, might induce tumorigenesis.

Some important factors and conditions regarding the role of the immune system in tumorigenesis are now becoming clear. First, most tumors are antigenic even if they are not immunogenic. Second, developing tumors are not ignored by the immune system. Many tumor cells express molecularly defined antigens that are recognized by cytotoxic and/or helper T lymphocytes. Moreover, manipulation of the immune system can lead to complete tumor eradication. However, the normal immune system is rarely a significant barrier to tumor growth and development. In most circumstances, tumors develop even in the presence of an apparently competent host immune system.

Tumors become clinically apparent only after a long process of tumorigenesis, the length of which may vary considerably among different tumors. However, the normal immune system should be vigilant from the early stages of tumorigenesis. Although early cellular events during tumorigenesis are not well understood, a strict clonality is maintained during the development of tumors. Some cells transform into tumor-like or precancerous cells. Although the host immune system should block the growth of such cells, they continue to grow and in time become overt tumors. Thus, it is important to understand the nature and characteristics of these precancerous cells. I use the terms "precancerous cells," "tumor-like cells," and "transformed cells" to indicate cells in the initial state of tumorigenesis.

The goal of this chapter is not to provide detailed accounts of immunological events in tumor immunology but to discuss the role of antigen-presenting dendritic cells (DCs), the most professional antigen-presenting cells (APCs), in tumorigenesis. The prospects for DC-based therapy for human tumors will also be discussed.

Dendritic Cells as Positive and Negative Regulators of Tumorigenesis

DCs are derived from CD34$^+$ hematopoietic progenitor cells (HPC) and are widely distributed in the body. They are highly heterogeneous with respect to their levels of activation and maturation. In addition, they have a wide variety of functions. DC progenitors, DC precursors, immature DCs, mature DCs, and exhausted DCs may be present in different tissues or in different compartments of the same tissue. From a functional perspective, DCs may be in any of several modes. In antigen-capturing mode, they recognize, capture, internalize, and process microbes, tumor cells, or their antigens (Ags). The capture and processing of Ags endow DCs with migratory capacity so that they leave the affected tissue, move to the lymphoid tissues via lymphatic vessels, and undergo maturation. In the lymph nodes, DCs are in Ag-presenting mode. They interact with lymphocytes in immunological synapses leading to the formation of Ag-specific lymphocytes.

Antigen presentation by DCs can also cause immune tolerance, which might be the main physiological role DCs in the steady state. Several factors might be responsible for determining whether the outcome of the immune response initiated by DCs is immunity or immune tolerance. The nature and dose of Ags, the affinity of Ags, tissue microenvironments, and the nature of the DCs to which the Ags were presented may determine the type of immune response.

As both immunogenic and tolerogenic DCs are present in situ, these cells are considered to be regulators of the immune response. DCs can act as both negative and positive modulators of immune reactions, even in tumor settings. Although DCs are considered to be antitumorigenic, they might also induce tumorigenesis. The putative antitumorigenic and tumorigenic effects of DCs are shown in Fig. 6.1. Some of the activities of DCs may be both antitumorigenic and tumorigenic. Cytokines and immune mediators produced by DCs may function in both these ways. Understanding the cellular basis of these functions in vivo is a challenging aspect of DC research.

In general, the detection of impaired APC functioning of DCs in tumor-bearing hosts, implicates DCs in tumorigenesis. Most of these APC functions are evaluated by checking the allostimulatory capacity of DCs. Although allostimulatory capacity is a nonspecific function of DCs, it does not encompass the tumor-associated antigen (TAA)-recognizing, -capturing, and -processing capacities of DCs. Moreover, DCs with increased allostimulatory capacity are not able to induce Ag-specific activation of T cells in all circumstances. It may not be possible to use TAAs to evaluate the functioning of DCs in tumor-bearing hosts, but studies reflecting the antigen-handling and T-cell stimulatory capacities of DCs in the context of tumor immunology are required to understand thoroughly the role of DCs in tumor immunology.

DCs are not a homogeneous cell population. They comprise several subtypes with distinct functional heterogeneity. The multiple of types of DCs may reflect the developmental characteristics of different precursor populations, or the phenotypes of DCs

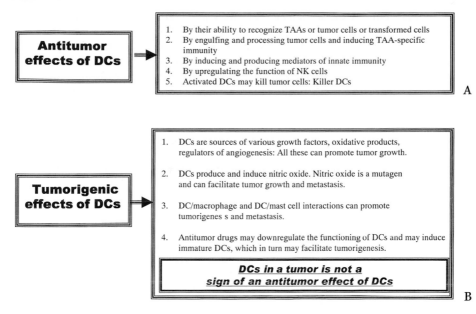

Antitumor effects of DCs

1. By their ability to recognize TAAs or tumor cells or transformed cells
2. By engulfing and processing tumor cells and inducing TAA-specific immunity
3. By inducing and producing mediators of innate immunity
4. By upregulating the function of NK cells
5. Activated DCs may kill tumor cells: Killer DCs

A

Tumorigenic effects of DCs

1. DCs are sources of various growth factors, oxidative products, regulators of angiogenesis: All these can promote tumor growth.

2. DCs produce and induce nitric oxide. Nitric oxide is a mutagen and can facilitate tumor growth and metastasis.

3. DC/macrophage and DC/mast cell interactions can promote tumorigenes s and metastasis.

4. Antitumor drugs may downregulate the functioning of DCs and may induce immature DCs, which in turn may facilitate tumorigenesis.

DCs in a tumor is not a sign of an antitumor effect of DCs

B

Fig. 6.1A,B. The putative tumorigenic and antitumor effects of dendritic cells (DCs). DCs have potent antitumor effects (A). However, DCs can also induce tumorigenesis under certain conditions (B)

might also be influenced by tissue microenvironments. Impaired functioning of immunogenic DCs may decrease the immune surveillance capacity of DCs leading to tumorigenesis. On the other hand, the increased functioning of tolerogenic DCs may not be beneficial for the tumor-bearing hosts, but instead may cause a flare-up of tumorigenesis. Thus, studies of DC subsets and their functions should be done in tumor-bearing hosts to understand the actual role of DCs in tumorigenesis.

In general, infiltration of DCs into tumor nodules, especially of mature DCs, has been considered to be a good prognostic marker. Evidence supporting this concept is accumulating: increased localization of DCs in tumors has been found to be correlated with a better prognosis. Based on this relationship, the administration of DCs to tumor-bearing hosts has become a general target of DC-based immune therapy for tumors. However, the following important facts must be borne in mind to make a proper evaluation of the role of DCs in tumor biology. Cells of the immune system, including DCs, are a source of growth factors, oxidative products, and regulators of angiogenesis, all of which might facilitate tumor growth (Fig. 6.1B). For example, granulocytes are required for the aggressive growth of some variants of ultraviolet radiation-induced tumors. Mast cells can also stimulate cancer growth under certain conditions. Oxidative products such as nitric oxide (NO) can serve as mutagens and facilitate tumor growth and metastasis, although NO can also kill tumor cells. Macrophages play several critical roles in tumor angiogenesis, including conversion of plasminogen to angiostatin. Immune system enhancement by tumor growth is especially common in hematopoietic tumors, where normal physiological networks of cytokine and cell-surface interactions become the driving force of tumor growth. Finally, the lymphocyte-specific genomic instability inherent in antibody and T-cell receptor gene rearrangements is a factor in the majority of lymphoid malignancies. Like granulocytes, mast cells, macrophages, and lymphocytes, DCs produce a variety of cytokines and chemokines and several immune modulators. They also induce several mediators from other cells of the immune system. However, a direct role for DCs in tumorigenesis has yet to be established.

On the other hand, DCs are the most potent APCs. They are responsible for the recognition and capture of Ags, including tumor cells, transformed cells, and precancerous cells. DCs are thought to induce an effective antitumor immunity by which the tumors should be eradicated from the tumor-bearing hosts. Naturally, when there is uncontrolled growth of tumors, impaired function of DCs is readily predicted. Several studies during the last 10 years have shown impaired function of DCs in tumor-bearing hosts. Furthermore, DCs in tumor microenvironments have shown decreased levels of maturation and activation. Finally, the introduction of DCs along with putative TAAs have resulted in the eradication or size reduction of tumors in most animal models. TAA-specific immunity has been also been traced in many of these cases. Moreover, injection of DCs along with products of tumor cells (a source of TAAs) has been shown in some animal models to protect against tumors during subsequent challenges with the same tumors. Some DCs expressing FasL are able to kill target cells in vitro. These DCs have been called "killer DCs." A population of DCs in situ has also been shown to express FasL, but the capacity of these DCs to destroy target cells or tumor cells has not been directly evaluated.

A therapeutic effect of DC-based therapy in human cancer has yet to be established, but the initial results of therapeutic trials inspire optimism. Although the above-mentioned discussion favors the notion that DCs may influence the course of tumors either positively or negatively, a more precise understanding of the role of DCs in specific tumors is required to bring DCs from the lab bench to the bedside. Although it is most important to learn whether DCs play any role in the initiation of tumorigenesis, this cannot be studied in several human tumors, so appropriate animal models are needed. Moreover, some tumors arise from a definite precancerous state, so the functioning of DCs needs to be studied both in precancerous tissues and during tumorigenesis. In addition, it is important to understand why uncontrolled growth of tumors occurs in spite of the existence of so-called functional DCs in situ and why anti-TAA specific immunity cannot be properly initiated in tumor-bearing hosts. As DCs have several functions, it is important to determine whether the defective functioning of DCs during tumorigenesis involves their immunogenic or tolerogenic roles.

DCs as Scanners of Tumor Cells In Vivo

As DCs are extremely divergent with respect to their phenotypes and functions, insights are needed into the role of DCs in tumorigenesis and their possible roles in tumor immune therapy. These can be explored by viewing a tumor as a kind of massive infection. As with a massive infection, persons suffering from tumors possess a huge quantity of cells that grow unrestrictedly in many sites in an organ or in different parts of the body. Tumorigenesis begins with the transformation of a normal

Requirement of a scanner in vivo for control of initiation and recurrence of tumors

1. A tumor is like a massive infection, and many tumor cells are present over the whole body.
2   Regeneration is a feature of all tumors, either at the primary site or in another location.
3   Antitumor therapy deletes the main tumor mass only.
4   There is a lack of surveillance for tumor cells in the whole body.
5   Even if tumor cells are detected, there is no means to eradicate them in vivo.

A

DCs as scanners for tumor cells in vivo

1. Widely distributed in the body in all tissues.
2. Can recognize, capture, and process tumor cells, transformed cells, or overt tumors.
3. Can activate cells of innate immunity such as NK cells and macrophages and produce type-1 interferon.
4. Able to induce adaptive immunity to TAAs.

B

Inability of DCs to properly scan for tumor cells

1. Impaired mobilization of DCs
2. Impaired recognition of tumor cells by DCs
3. Lack of expression of TAAs or sequestration of TAAs within tumors
4. DCs may not recognize TAAs because of mutations
5. Apoptosis of DCs due to engulfment of tumor cells
6. Inability of DCs to process tumor cells and impaired migration of DCs to lymphoid tissues
7. Impaired formation of TAA-specific lymphocytes
8. Defective migration and impaired survival of TAA-specific lymphocytes at tumor tissues
9. Extensive tumor burden making DCs incapable of handling tumor load

C

Fig. 6.2A–C. DCs as immunlolgical scanners for tumor cells. A Scanner-like DCs are essential for host defense in the context of tumor immunity. B The expected roles of DCs as scanners for tumor cells in vivo. The appearance of tumors means that DCs could not act properly as scanners for tumor cells. The underlying causes are summarized (C). *NK*, natural killer; *TAA*, tumor-associated antigen

cell to a tumor-like cell, which can also be called a precancerous or transformed cell. The tumor-like cells multiply over time, but it is not clear whether they grow unrestrictedly or whether they become tumors only after overcoming many blockades in vivo. When an apparent tumor develops, and the goal is to treat that tumor. Tumor therapy includes the use of antitumor medications or ablation of the tumor mass by surgery. However, these therapeutic approaches cannot eliminate all tumor cells. Even if the main bulk of the tumor is removed from the host, some tumor cells remain. Moreover, new tumor cells will be generated in the same host. Thus, the major problem with tumorigenesis is the recurrence or progression of tumors. How can this aspect of tumorigenesis be addressed? A proper scanning system for tumor cells in vivo is needed. DCs may act like such a scanner owing to their ability detect tumors or tumor-like cells in vivo. The reasons that a tumor scanning system is needed are listed in Fig. 6.2A. DCs may be one of the best in vivo scanners for tumorigenesis (Fig. 6.2B): they are mobile; they can recognize microbes and their antigens and abnormal cells (dead cells, transformed cells, and perhaps tumor cells); and they are able to internalize those objects and induce an immune response against them. Most importantly, investigations during the last three decades have provided ways to manipulate the activities of DCs both in vitro and in vivo. DCs in vivo act as sentinels of the immune system by scanning whether any cells are undergoing malignant transformation. The recognition of transformed cells or tumor cells is vital for subsequent antitumor immunity. However, DCs apparently are not always able to do this scanning function properly, which leads to the accumulation of tumor cells in vivo, that is, the initiation of tumorigenesis (Fig. 6.2C). The development of an overt tumor indicates that the scanning system has failed for some reason. As tumor cells grow unrestrictedly over time, they may produce mediators that downregulate the scanning capacity of DCs, causing further development of tumors. How can this scanning system be made viable and effective in vivo? It is premature to speculate about this until we understand better the condition of DCs in the precancerous state. How can the DC-based scanning system be revitalized after the growth of visible tumors in vivo? At present, it is not clearly known whether the administration of activated DCs would accomplish this revitalization.

Putative Roles of DCs During the Initiation of Carcinogenesis

The possible roles of DCs in the initiation and progression of tumorigenesis are summarized in Fig. 6.3. DCs with impaired functioning, defective activation, and distorted maturation have been identified in the peripheral blood and in tumor tissues of patients with tumors and in tumors of experimental model animals. These findings

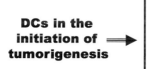

DCs in the initiation of tumorigenesis ⟹

1. Effect of DCs on the expression and activity of antioncogenes?
2. Impact of DC-induced mediators on oncogenes and anti-oncogenes
4. DCs maintaining chronic inflammation, which may cause genetic instability and tumorigenesis.
5. Nitric oxide and oncogenic modulators produced by DCs
6. Therapy that may downregulate DC functioning and make DCs incapable of acting as potent APCs
7. Inadequate support by DCs of cells of innate immunity such as NK cells and macrophages.
8. Lack of type-1-1FN producing DCs in tissue
9. Impaired induction of antitumor immunity by DCs

A

DCs in the progression of tumorigenesis ⟹

Existence of visible tumors means that the scanning capacity of DCs for tumor cells is either impaired or lost

1. Tumor-derived factors may further downregulate DC functioning and may help the progression of tumors:

a) Impaired activation of DCs
b) Defective production of progenitors and precursors of DCs
c) Defective activation and maturation of DCs
d) Defective survival of DCs and activated CTLs

B

Fig. 6.3A,B. Putative roles of Dcs in the initiation and progression of tumorigenesis. During the initiation of tumorigenesis, DCs might have divergent roles. Many DC-derived factors may induce tumorigenesis. Also, impaired functioning of DCs may underlie the initiation of tumorigenesis (**A**). The existence of an overt tumor means, that the immune surveillance mechanism has failed, and DCs could not scan properly for the tumor cells. An impairment of different functions of DCs might be responsible (**B**). *APC*, antigen-presenting cell; *CTL*, cytotoxic T lymphocyte; *IFN*, interferon

have led to the conclusion that defectively functioning DCs play a role in tumorigenesis. However, that appears to be an oversimplification of a complex issue. To evaluate their phenotypes and functions, DCs have been enriched or isolated from tumor-bearing patients or from experimental animal models of tumors. Most of these subjects had suffered from tumors for a quite long period. In fact, patients with established tumors show defective functioning of almost all types of cells of the immune system, which mainly reflects the impact of tumorigenesis on the host immune system. Moreover, antitumor therapy may also suppress the functioning of the cells of the immune system, including that of DCs. Thus, it remains to be established whether impaired functioning of DCs induces tumorigenesis or whether their impaired functioning is an effect of tumorigenesis. Although the second possibility is very likely in clinical contexts, the roles of DCs in the initiation of tumorigenesis deserve special attention. The nature and functions of DCs during the initiation of tumorigenesis cannot be studied for most tumors, mainly because most human tumors lack a well-established precancerous state. Many cells transform into cells with abnormal features on a daily basis in vivo, and such transformations represent a normal cellular event in living organisms. Changes in the tissue microenvironment and immunological stress on the host are also capable of inducing such cellular alterations. Reticuloendothelial cells usually clear these transformed cells to maintain homeostasis. Under certain conditions, some of these transformed cells become premalignant cells or tumor cells and continue to grow in an unrestricted fashion. The products of a set of genes called oncogenes influence the malignant transformation of cells. In contrast, the antitumor effects of the products of anti-oncogenes counter the tumorigenic potentials of oncogenes. The role of DCs in maintaining the balance between the activities of the products of oncogenes and those of anti-oncogenes has not been adequately addressed. However, it is known that inflammatory and other changes in the tissue microenvironment influence the expression of the products of oncogenes and anti-oncogenes.

As a part of the host defense activity, the invasion of tissues by microbes is followed by their recognition, capture, and processing by DCs in the affected tissue, which then migrate to lymphoid tissue to induce the expansion and activation of clonally selected microbe-specific cytotoxic T lymphocytes (CTLs). These CTLs migrate to the tissue of microbial invasion and destroy the microbe-infected cells. If, owing to the impaired functioning of DCs, an infection is not completely eradicated but becomes chronic, the infected cells and tissues undergo repeated destruction and regeneration. This process may lead to the production of cells with malignant potential. In addition, nitric oxide and other DC-derived factors may be tumorigenic for the host.

In addition to these tumorigenic potentials, DCs may play a dominant role during the initiation of tumorigenesis because they regulate the functioning of two of the most important cells of the innate immune system, natural killer (NK) cells and macrophages. When cells undergo malignant transformation, NK cells should come forward to eliminate them. It is now evident that there is cross talk between NK cells and DCs. If the functioning of NK cells is impaired by the impairment of DC function, tumor cells or transformed cells may not be cleared by the cells of the innate immune system. Moreover, DCs and macrophages are both differentiated from CD34$^+$ HPCs. If proper development of macrophages is hampered by the skewing of their precursors to DCs, innate immunity may be compromised. The role of cytokines and other mediators in the development of DCs and macrophages and their interrelationship has recently started to be unmasked, and new information is likely to enrich our understanding of these phenomena.

Recently, a precursor population of DCs was shown to be a potent producer of type-1 interferon (IFN). These cells are called natural IFN-producing cells (NIPCs). In addition, it is now evident that almost all subsets of DCs can produce type-1 IFN in vitro. Type-I IFN acts as a bridge between the innate and adaptive immune systems, as it is thought to provide the danger signals when the tissue microenvironment is altered by microbial infection or inflammatory changes. Impaired production of type-1 IFN by DCs would impair the danger signaling system that induces the immune response and would thus provide an opportunity for chronic infection, inflammation, and tumorigenesis.

In addition to these DC functions in innate immunity, DCs have the most vital role in the induction of adaptive immunity. As sentinels of the immune system, DCs recognize, internalize and process TAAs from transformed cells to induce TAA-specific immunity in vivo. The failure of DCs to induce effective antitumor immunity in situ may result in the uncontrolled growth of a tumor.

Putative Roles of DCs During the Progression of Tumorigenesis

Irrespective of the mechanism underlying the conversion of normal cells to tumor cells, the major problem in clinics is the uncontrolled growth of tumors in vivo. This is most evident when an overt tumor is diagnosed in a clinical setting. While it is true that several cells are converted into tumor-like cells on a daily basis, clinically apparent tumors do not normally result from these cellular changes. Even in immunocompromised hosts, only selective tumors are detected and tumors of multiple organs are never found in these patients under any conditions. Once a tumor is present in a host, it is readily understood that the DCs of the host failed to successfully scan for the tumor cells in vivo, leading to the development of the visible tumor. Some possible factors that might underlie the progression of tumors are listed in Fig. 6.3B. Developing tumors can downregulate DC functions by producing various factors. Impaired functioning of DCs, their defective maturation, a distorted migratory capacity, and defective production and induction of cytokines by DCs might compromise their antitumor effect. These conditions worsen further if the patients receive antitumor therapy incorporating drugs that downregulate DC function. Thus, once a tumor has developed in a host, DC functioning will be further downregulated, which might allow more precancerous lesions to become visible tumors.

Nature of Dendritic Cell Defects During Tumorigenesis

Circumstantial evidence strongly suggests that, either directly or indirectly, alone or in concert with other cells of the immune system, DCs play an important role in the initiation and progression of tumors. Most of the cellular events relating to DCs in tumorigenesis are not yet clear. However, it is certain that the functions of DCs are variably modified in different tumors. Functional abnormalities of DCs relevant to tumorigenesis are diagrammed in Fig. 6.4.

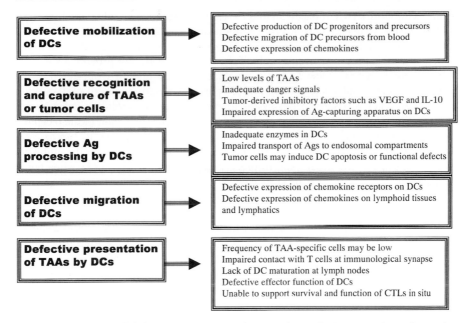

Defective mobilization of DCs	Defective production of DC progenitors and precursors Defective migration of DC precursors from blood Defective expression of chemokines
Defective recognition and capture of TAAs or tumor cells	Low levels of TAAs Inadequate danger signals Tumor-derived inhibitory factors such as VEGF and IL-10 Impaired expression of Ag-capturing apparatus on DCs
Defective Ag processing by DCs	Inadequate enzymes in DCs Impaired transport of Ags to endosomal compartments Tumor cells may induce DC apoptosis or functional defects
Defective migration of DCs	Defective expression of chemokine receptors on DCs Defective expression of chemokines on lymphoid tissues and lymphatics
Defective presentation of TAAs by DCs	Frequency of TAA-specific cells may be low Impaired contact with T cells at immunological synapse Lack of DC maturation at lymph nodes Defective effector function of DCs Unable to support survival and function of CTLs in situ

Fig. 6.4. The nature of defects in various populations of DCs during tumorigenesis. During tumorigenesis, about all types of functions of DCs might be impaired. There might be impaired mobilization of DCs in the tissue or induction of TAA-specific immunity in vivo. Many tumor-derived factors might even compromise the survival and functioning of DCs

Defective Mobilization of DCs in the Tumor Microenvironment

When tumor-like cells express TAAs, DCs and possibly other cells of the innate immune system should mobilize at the site of the transformed cells, leading to their eradication and the induction of TAA-specific immunity in vivo. Mobilization of sufficient numbers of immature DCs is dependent on various factors such as (1) development of DC progenitors in the bone marrow and (2) migration of DC precursors from the bone marrow to the blood and then from the blood to the tissues. In addition, some DC precursors in tissues may also differentiate into immature DCs, depending on the local microenvironment. Although cells of the innate immune system, such as granulocytes, NK cells, and macrophages, may destroy the evolving tumor-like cells, the mobilization of DCs is essential for the induction of TAA-specific immunity. Mobilization of DC progenitors and DC precursors from the bone marrow and blood to the tissue of localization of the tumor-like cells requires the expression of chemokines in that tissue, the presence of inflammatory factors, and the expression of chemokine receptors on DC populations. After the mobilization of DC precursors, they should be converted to immature DCs according to their lineage commitment and the availability of cytokines in the tissue. For example, high levels of IL-6 in the local tissue may direct these cells toward a macrophage lineage, whereas granulocyte-macrophage colony-stimulating factor (GM-CSF) would ensure the transition to immature DCs. If plasmacytoid DCs in the tissue secrete substantial amounts of type-1 IFN, that may permit proper mobilization of DCs in the affected tissues. Even after tumor-like cells are present, DCs may not be mobilized in full vigor at the tissue of localization of the tumor cells if the tumor cells do not provide a so-called danger signal, that is, if few TAAs are produced or they remain sequestered in the tumor-like cells. Inadequate production of cytokines or expression of certain other relevant proteins in tissues harboring the tumor cells may also result in defective DC mobilization. Defective expression of chemokines in tissues and chemokine receptors on DCs may disrupt the normal mobilization of DCs in response to tumor cells. Understanding these cellular events will provide additional insight into the mobilization of DCs in normal tissues and in precancerous tissue. For example, when hepatocytes from a cirrhotic liver or gastric epithelial cells from a stomach with gastritis transform into premalignant cells in situ, these cells might not be able to provide adequate signals, including danger signals, for the mobilization of DCs. Even the local microenvironment might be distorted in these tissues in such a way that the signals from the local tissue are disrupted. This may also be true of DC mobilization in the lungs of heavy smokers. Thus, even if there is an adequate pool of DC precursors in the bone marrow and blood, these DC precursors might not be able to mobilize in the liver, stomach, or lung tissues, where the transformed cells continue to grow and where additional cells are undergoing alteration. The mobilization capacity of DCs would be further impaired if the expression of chemokines or their receptors by the DCs was already impaired because of the prolonged pathological processes of the premalignant state. Thus, tumor-like hepatocytes in patients with liver cirrhosis or gastric epithelial cells in patients with gastritis or inflamed lung cells in heavy smokers might not be able to induce the proper signals for DC mobilization. The alteration of tissue architecture in these premalignant states may also obstruct DC mobilization by blocking migration of DC precursors through vessels and by inducing the abnormal expression of chemokines. These events have not been shown experimentally, but they should be seriously considered when designing a DC-based therapy for tumors.

This scenario is not only applicable to the induction of immune responses to so-called putative premalignant cells or tumor-like cells, but it is equally valid in the context of developing tumors. When a tumor attains a considerable size, it becomes more important that huge numbers of DCs be mobilized at the site of tumor for the induction of adaptive immunity against cancer. In these circumstances, the mobilization of not only DCs is important, but also of other immunocytes, including TAA-specific CTLs, which are essential for the eradication of the tumor.

The following events and circumstances affect the mobilization of DC precursors during the initial stage of tumorigenesis.

1. Alteration in the rate of hematopoiesis in precancerous tissue and in subjects harboring tumor-like cells and, especially, of production of multipotential $CD34^+$ HPCs in the bone marrow.
2. Phenotypic alteration of DC progenitors and their migration to the peripheral blood.
3. Availability of danger signals from tumor-like cells and the microenvironment of the tissue harboring the tumor-like cells.

4. The intensity and the magnitude of expression of chemokines and chemokine receptors on blood vessels, tissues, DC precursors, and immature DCs.
5. Availability and nature of cytokines in and around the tumor-like cells, including the presence of cytokines inhibitory to DC functioning, such as IL-10, vascular endothelial growth factors, and prostaglandins.
6. The physical barrier provided by the capsule of cancer cells. For example, in cirrhotic liver and encapsulated HCC, the capsule may be a formidable barrier to the entry of DCs.
7. The subsets of DCs mobilized at the site of transformed cells. Different DC subsets perform different types of functions, and some DC subsets are not designed for capturing and processing antigens.

Defective Recognition and Capture of TAAs by DCs

The malignant transformation of cells is a common event in vivo, but in most cases, an overt tumor does not develop because several anti-oncogenic factors block the initial transformation of normal cells to tumor-like cells. Even if cells are transformed to tumor-like cells, cells of the innate immune system destroy and dispose of those tumor-like cells to block the progression to an overt tumor. Nevertheless, despite the activities of these factors, tumors develop and grow unrestrictedly in different sites of the body.

During the initial phase of tumorigenesis, DCs get signals from the tissue harboring transformed or premalignant cells or malignant cells to mobilize at the affected organs. After the DCs are appropriately mobilized at the affected tissues, the next immunological event is the recognition of the so-called transformed cells or malignant cells by the DCs. In order to recognize microbes, DCs use a group of receptors called pattern-recognition receptors, such as toll-like receptors (TLRs). However, it is not clear how DCs recognize potential tumor cells, transformed cells, or malignant cells. The expression of ligands for TLRs has not been studied in tumor cells. So called danger signals provided by the tissue microenvironment may help DCs to recognize tumor cells or transformed cells. The inflammatory cytokines in the tissue microenvironment may be a source of these danger signals.

Although the mechanism for recognition of tumor-like cells by immature DCs is not clear, DCs are equipped with potent apparatuses capable of internalizing Ags and cells. DCs use macropinocytosis, Fcγ and Fcε receptors, and lectin receptors for internalization purposes. The levels of expression of these receptors on DCs have not been evaluated in tissues harboring tumor-like cells, so it is not known whether the expression of the Ag-internalization apparatuses is compromised in a precancerous or tumor microenvironment. Naturally, it is also unknown whether defective engulfment of transformed cells by DCs underlies the defective antigen-specific immune response in these situations.

When DCs are assigned to capture growing tumor cells, many added factors could make antigen capture more difficult. DCs might take in apoptotic cells by using the CD51/vitronectin receptor αvβ3 or CD36/thrombospondin receptors. The expression of these receptors on DCs in the cancer microenvironment, however, has not been explored.

Although little information on DC functioning in the microenvironment of transformed cells is available, the tumor microenvironment is usually hostile to the proper functioning of DCs. Tumors produce a variety of cytokines and mediators that may block DC functioning. One of the major limitations of our understanding of the capture of TAAs and cancer cells by DCs is that it is completely unknown whether DCs internalize all types of TAAs or only some types, because several TAAs may be present in a particular tumor.

Even if the DCs in the tumor microenvironment possess a potent antigen-capturing apparatus, important questions include how and under what conditions DCs can take up TAAs or tumor cells in vivo. The capture of Ags in a microenvironment with inhibitory cytokines or factors such as IL-10 or vascular endothelial growth factor may not result in the induction of an immune response against the captured Ags. It is important to study the viability of DCs after they have internalized apoptotic tumor cells. Engulfment of tumor cells may induce apoptosis of DCs. Finally, even after the tumor cells or TAAs have been engulfed, DCs may just ignore these cells, owing to a lack of danger signals from them.

In summary, how do DCs recognize transformed cells or tumor cells? If TLRs are involved in this process, the identification of ligands for TLRs in tumor-like cells and in overt malignant cells is important. The ligands may be highly variable, depending on the nature and genesis of the transformed cells. For example, if microbial infections underlie the pathogenesis of the tumor cells, then microbe-related TLRs on DCs might be involved in their recognition. However, this is a black hole in our understanding of the recognition of tumors and their associated particles by DCs.

The following points regarding the recognition and capture of tumor cells or transformed cells by DCs might be relevant in the context of tumor immunity.

1. The presence of danger signals in the tissue harboring transformed cells or TAAs and tumors.
2. The levels of expression and the regulation of various antigen-engulfing apparatuses on blood DCs in the precancerous state or on tissue DCs after their mobilization to the cancerous tissues.
3. The survival of DCs after engulfing tumor-like cells or tumors. The cancer microenvironment, including the presence of inhibitory factors such as IL-10, vascular endothelial growth factor, and macrophage colony-stimulating factor, is important in this regard.
4. Alterations of the functional capacities of DCs after internalization of tumor cells.

Defective Processing of Tumor Cells or TAAs by DCs

A TAA-specific immune response depends on the processing of transformed cells, TAAs, or tumor cells by DCs. Both DCs and macrophages are able to capture and internalize antigens or cells, but the induction of a primary immune response is mediated by DCs, not by macrophages. The main factor underlying this limitation has to do with the intracellular migration and processing of the engulfed TAAs or Ags derived from the tumor cells. Macrophages, although able to internalize antigens or cells, are unable to transmit the internalized antigens to major histocompatibility complex (MHC) class I or class II compartments. In contrast, DCs can load the internalized antigens into an endosomal compartment, where they induce the formation of an MHC class II compartment (MIIC). The migration of these MIICs to the DC surface allows the DCs to express the Ags along with self-MHC molecules. It is still unclear whether transformed cells or their antigens are properly programmed to MIICs, and it is also unknown whether an MIIC complex containing tumor-derived antigens moves to the DC surface for alignment with self-MHC. A similar sequence of events may occur during the transmission of Ags to MHC class I compartments in DCs.

To understand the relationship between antigen processing and the induction of antitumor immunity by DCs, the following points should be considered.

1. Release of TAAs from transformed cells or tumor cells in DCs
2. Migration of TAAs to endosomal compartments and MIICs in DCs in the tumor microenvironment
3. Migration of MIICs to the surface of DCs in the tumor microenvironment. The role of inhibitory cytokines needs to be studied in this regard.
4. Alteration of Ag processing in DCs engulfing tumor-like cells, tumor cells, or TAAs.
5. The role of the tumor microenvironment in regulating these processes.

Defective Migration of DCs in the Tumor Microenvironment

If DC precursors are able to mobilize properly in tumor-harboring tissues, if they can capture and process tumor-like cells or TAAs adequately, and if TAAs are expressed on the surfaces of DCs along with self-MHC molecules, then these DCs are now ready to migrate to lymphoid tissues for the induction of an Ag-specific immune response. In the usual circumstances, the uptake and successful processing of Ags through endosomal compartments lead to the activation of the DCs, which is manifested by the upregulation of costimulatory molecules such as CD86, CD80, and CD40. At the same time, the activity of the antigen-capturing apparatus of the DCs and the expression of CC chemokine receptor (CCR) 6 is downregulated.

Although DCs with defective maturation and activation status have been detected in tumor tissues, direct experimental evidence showing that this defective state was caused by the intake of tumor-like cells or tumor cells by the DCs is lacking. The impaired activation and maturation of DCs in tumor tissues may be induced by tumor-derived factors or by inhibitory cytokines localized in the tumor microenvironment because factors such as IL-10 and vascular endothelial growth factor block the activation and maturation of DCs in vitro, and these factors are abundant in most tumor microenvironments. Thus, in spite of the production of a set of immunogenic DCs in vivo after internalization of tumor cells or TAAs, huge numbers of tolerogenic DCs may form in situ as a result of environmental factors. Consistent with this, presentation of TAAs by tolerogenic DCs would lead to immune tolerance of, not immunity to, TAAs.

Even if DCs undergo maturation and activation in cancer microenvironments, the most important step is the alteration of the expression of chemokine receptors on maturating DCs from the immature to the mature type. Immature DCs express CCR6 and mobilize to the tissues in response to a call from macrophage inflammatory protein (MIP)-3α, which is expressed in the tissues. However, when Ags, along with MHC molecules, are expressed by DCs, they are thought to downregulate the expression of CCR6, followed by increased expression of CCR7. This CCR7 expression is related to the activation and migration of these DCs to secondary lymphoid organs. Ligands for CCR7 should be expressed on lymphatic vessel cells at the same time. Studies have shown abundant expression of MIP-3α on parenchymal cells in cancers such as pancreatic and breast cancers. Our research group has also documented increased MIP-3α levels in the sera of patients with HCC, which might have originated from the cancer tissues. Thus, although the expression of MIP-3α should be downregulated for the induction of a TAA-specific immune response, that was not the case with these cancers.

The following points deserve serious consideration to gain insight into the low antitumor immunity in tumor settings.

1. The expression of cytokines such as IL-10, vascular endothelial growth factor, and IL-6 in the cancer microenvironment. These cytokines and modulators can influence the functioning of DCs at different levels of Ag presentation.
2. The expression of CCR6 and CCR7 on DCs in the cancer microenvironment and their ligands in cancer and lymphatic tissues.

For antitumor immunity to be induced, evasion of DCs from the cancer microenvironment must occur. DCs bearing the immunogenic epitopes of TAAs should leave the tumor tissues and enter the lymphatic vessels to move to the secondary lymphoid organs. This movement is dependent not only on the expression of CCR7 on DCs but also on the expression of MIP-3β and secondary lymphoid-tissue chemokines (SLCs) on lymphatic and lymphoid tissues.

Expression of CCR7 on DCs has been shown to be downregulated in certain malignancies, but these experiments were done on DCs isolated from noncancerous tissues. The expression of CCR7 on DCs from cancer or lymphoid tissues needs to be studied.

Defective Presentation of TAAs by DCs in the Lymphoid Tissue

Very few studies have addressed antigen presentation by DCs in the lymphoid tissues in the context of tumors. For this reason, the phenotypes and maturation status of DCs in the secondary lymphoid organs of patients with tumors should be explored. However, this is a very difficult task. It is impossible to locate TAA-specific DC–T cell interactions and TAA-unrelated DC–T cell interactions in the lymph nodes because the frequencies of activated T cells are low in lymph nodes from patients with tumors. However, such studies have not been done in patients with early malignancies. Thus, it is uncertain whether the lack of activated DCs in cancer tissues is due to a generalized defect in advanced cancer patients or whether it reflects some immune regulatory defects of these patients to TAA. The following points should be considered regarding Ag presentation in the lymph nodes in the context of tumor immunology.

1. Frequencies of activated T cells and activated DCs in secondary lymphoid organs, especially during the early stage of cancers and in precancerous patients.
2. Expression of maturation and activation markers on DCs from lymphoid tissues.
3. Functional capacities of T cells and DCs isolated from cancer nodules.
4. Production of cytokines and mediators that may inhibit immune response.

Dysfunction of Mature DCs in Tumor Tissues

In principle, the role of DCs ends after they interact with lymphocytes and following presentation of TAAs to T lymphocytes in immunological synapses in the lymphoid tissues. When the T lymphocytes are activated in the lymph nodes in an antigen-specific fashion, the DCs undergo terminal maturation. The fate of these terminal DCs is not clear. They may undergo apoptosis, or they may be killed by the effector lymphocytes that they induced.

However, although DCs with maturation and activation markers can be detected in tissues, they are very few in malignant tissues. It is unknown how mature DCs accumulate in the peripheral tissues, but this is an extremely important event in the context of tumor immunity. Several hypotheses have been proposed regarding the localization of mature DCs in tissues, but experimental evidence on the molecular and cellular mechanisms underlying the localization of mature DCs in the peripheral tissue is lacking. The following points deserve attention:

1. Immature DCs in the peripheral tissues may undergo maturation at the local tissue by default. After Ag capture, they might not be able to migrate to the lymphoid tissues owing to defective expression of chemokines or their receptors. These DCs may acquire a mature phenotype as an effect of local cytokines. If this scenario is accurate, then these DCs do not present Ags to T lymphocytes because clonally selected Ag-specific T lymphocytes are detected in the lymphoid organs, but not in the peripheral tissues. It is important to consider whether these Ag-nonspecific DCs are functional.

2. These mature DCs may have come from the lymphoid tissues after presenting Ags to T lymphocytes in the immunological synapses. In the lymphoid tissues, DCs and lymphocytes make a very strong bridge with the help of several adhesion molecules. When the activated lymphocytes leave the lymph nodes and migrate to the peripheral tissues, the DCs may accompany them.

Very few mature DCs have been localized in tumor tissues, although higher numbers of mature DCs are detected in the noncancerous tissues near the tumors. To gain insight into the nature of different DC populations in tumors, our research group localized DCs by using immunohistochemical methods to check the expression of HLA DR, S100 antigen, and CD83 in patients with HCC and also in patients with liver cirrhosis, a precancerous state. Almost no CD83-positive mature DCs were detected in the cancerous tissue of HCC patients, but many such DCs were detected in precancerous cirrhotic nodules. It is interesting to note that DCs expressing HLA DR and S100 protein were seen with equal frequency in both cancer nodules and noncancerous cirrhotic nodules.

Some investigators have shown a relationship between the frequencies of DCs in the tissues and tumor prognosis. The major limitation of these studies is the methodology used to identify the DCs. In most of these studies, DCs were detected by their expression of S100 or HLA DR, and few studies used CD83 as a marker for DCs. Dr. Hart and his colleagues at Mater Medical Research Institute, Australia reported that two monoclonal antibodies react with mature DCs, but very few clinical studies have used these antibodies to define mature DCs in tissues. In vitro studies have also shown very few mature DCs in tumor tissues collected from various clinical and experimental samples.

What is the function of mature DCs in the tumor microenvironment? These DCs do not participate in the recognition, capture, processing, or presentation of Ags, which means that they are not designed to act as APCs. Although it is difficult to precisely define their roles, these DCs may be important for performing some effector function of the immune response. Activated CTLs and other activated T cells in the cancer microenvironment must survive to perform their functions, and several cytokines are required to ensure their survival. Mature DCs may perform an essential role in the survival and functioning of CTLs in cancer tissues by secreting a wide variety of cytokines.

Why are the frequencies of mature DCs low in cancer tissues? As the formation, migration, and function of these DCs in tissues are yet to be explored, no data are available from which to formulate a hypothesis on this elusive matter at this time. However, one might assume that mature DCs cannot survive in the cancer microenvironment. In fact, factors derived from cancer tissues have been shown to block the maturation of DCs in vitro in several instances. Nevertheless, the following questions and considerations are important in the context of the localization of mature DCs in cancer tissues.

1. How do mature DCs accumulate in cancer tissues or their adjacent tissues? Are they produced in those areas or do they come to the tumor tissues with the activated T cells from the lymphoid tissues?
2. Very few mature DCs are seen in peripheral blood of either controls or cancer patients. It is important to ascertain the source of mature DCs in the peripheral blood.
3. Chemokines are required for mobilization of mature DCs in cancer tissues. MIP-3β is required for the migration of mature DCs to the lymphoid tissues, but it is not known which chemokines are required for the migration of mature DCs to the cancer tissues.
4. Why are there very few mature DCs in the cancer microenvironment? Is the cancer microenvironment hostile to the survival of mature DCs? Can mature DCs not be produced there? Or is the migration of mature DCs from lymphoid tissues hampered in tumors.
5. What is the relationship between mature DCs and NK cells and between mature DCs and $CD8^+$ CTLs? Both NK cells and Ag-specific CTLs may kill mature DCs in tumor tissues.
6. What is the function of mature DCs in cancer tissues? Although these DCs express CD83, a marker of DC maturation, there is a paucity of information regarding their function. The bulk of DCs from tumor tissues exhibit impaired functioning, but no one has studied specifically the functioning of mature DCs from tumor tissues.

Localization and Characterization of DCs in Tumors

Introduction

DCs perform a variety of functions in vivo. Although the main functions of DCs are to recognize, process, and present antigens to T lymphocytes, they also have many other functions. They produce a variety of cytokines and mediators, including type-

1 IFN, make cross talk with NK cells, and perform many effector functions such as the killing of target cells. In the initial chapters of this book, I discussed how DCs may play a role in the initiation and progression of tumorigenesis, and how tumorigenesis can affect the functioning of DCs. Although intensive studies are required to develop proper insights into these problems, the ultimate goal is very clear-cut. First, it is necessary to evaluate whether DCs are functioning properly in the context of tumorigenesis. Next, it is necessary to evaluate whether manipulation of the functioning of DCs in tumor-bearing hosts can block the occurrence, progression, and complications of tumors. The first can be accomplished by evaluating antitumor immunity in situ. Whether antitumor immunity is present can be inferred from the extent and nature of tumor-specific T-lymphocyte responses in tumor-bearing hosts. The survival of the tumor-bearing host would also imply some degree of immunity. To this end, researchers have tried to locate DCs or DC-like cells in tumors and in other tissues of tumor-bearing hosts. Some of these studies have also determined the phenotypes and functions of the DCs from these subjects. The results of these studies will provide the means for addressing the second problem regarding the utility of DC-based therapy for tumors.

Localization of DCs in Human Tumors

Although immunohistochemical approaches are best for identifying DCs in situ, it is impossible to detect all types of DCs in tissue sections. DCs are highly heterogeneous regarding their expression of surface Ags, and there is no known marker that is expressed on all different types of DCs.

The most commonly applied markers for DCs in human tissues identify HLA class II molecules and their associated invariant chains, expressed in high density on the cell surface of DCs. Many anti-HLA class II molecules react with DCs in frozen sections and also in embedded fixed sections. However, these antibodies also react with macrophages, B cells, endothelial cells, and other associated activated cells, including T cells and epithelial cells.

The S100 family of intracytoplasmic calcium-binding proteins have traditionally been used to demonstrate dendritic populations such as Langerhans cells and interdigitating DCs in the lymph nodes. The specificity of staining is low because many other types of cells, such as lymphoid, nerve, and fat- and carbohydrate-storing cells, and melanocytes, also express S100 protein. As other DC markers are now available, it is apparent that S100 protein is expressed by only a subset of DCs. Although DCs contain homodimeric S100β with two β subunits, neural tissue contains heterodimeric S100 αβ subunits indicating a possibility of cross reaction.

CD68 antigen has been found to be expressed on some DCs, but it is basically a marker for macrophages. CD68 is also expressed on developing myeloid cells and on various other tumor cells.

Some immune accessory molecules, such as CD40, CD80, and CD86, and the adhesion molecules CD11c, ICAM-1, and ICAM-3, may be present on DCs from various tissues, but the sensitivity and specificity of these markers are too low for them to be used to detect DCs. Moreover, many cells, especially those that are situated in proximity to DCs in the tissues also express some of these markers. Antigens such as CD1a are expressed by some subsets of DCs, for example, skin LCs.

Table 6.1. Localized DCs and their implications

Tumors	Implications
Less in tumor	
Oral	Few in tumors
Head and Neck	Rare in tumors
Oropharynx	Less in tumors
Salivary glands	Few in tumors
Arsenical skin	Less in tumors
Basal cells	Less in tumors
Cervix	Less in tumors
Hepatoma	Almost nil in cancer nodules
Melanoma	Decreased DCs in tumors
Skin tumors	Less in tumors
Immature phenotype	
Thyroid	DCs with immature phenotype
Breast	Immature DCs in tumor
Good prognosis	
endometrial	LC infiltration-favorable prognosis
Larynx	Favorable prognosis
Nasopharyngeal	Related to good prognosis
Oral tongue	Related to prognosis
Cervix	Related to good prognosis
Esophageal	Improved prognosis
Gastric	Improved prognosis
Lung	Marked improved prognosis
Prostate	Improved prognosis
Unrelated to prognosis	
Oral squamous	No relation to prognosis
Bronchoalveolar	No effect

LC, Langehans cell

Newer molecules of interest for the study of DCs in situ include CD83, RelB, which is a member of the nuclear factor (NF)-κB family of transcription factors, CMRF-44, and CMRF-56. CD83 is thought to be unique to monocyte-derived cultured-blood DCs, but recently CD83-positive DCs have been located in tissue sections, even in fixed tissue sections, by some investigators.

Fascin, a 55-kDa actin-binding protein, is expressed on DCs from different sources. However, the usefulness of fascin as a tissue marker of DCs is limited owing to its low specificity and its expression on capillary endothelial cells.

DCs have been detected in tumor tissues from several malignancies, such as basal skin cell carcinoma, breast cancer, nasopharyngeal cancers, oropharyngeal cancers, laryngeal cancers, oral cancers, cancers of the salivary glands, cancers of the head and neck, bronchoalveolar carcinoma, cervical carcinoma, endometrial carcinoma, gastric cancer, hepato cellular carcinoma, Hodgkin disease, lung cancer, melanoma, prostate cancer, and thyroid cancer (Table 6.1). This list grows day by day. In general, most studies have shown that DCs are fewer in tumor tissue compared with noncancerous tissues and normal tissues of the same organs. For example, in patients with HCC,

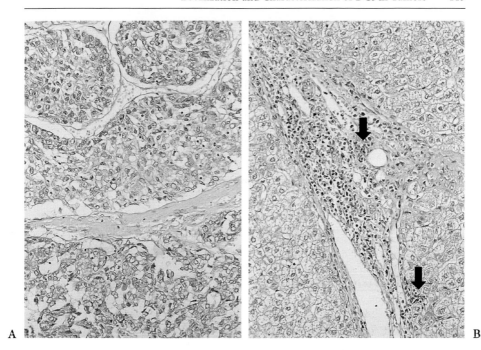

A   B

Fig. 6.5A,B. **A** Almost no CD83-positive mature DCs were found in cancer nodules in livers from patients with hepatocellular carcinoma. However, mature DCs expressing CD83 (reddish signals) were seen in the live tissue of patients with liver cirrhosis, a precancerous state of hepatocellular carcinoma (**B**). *Arrows*, mature DC. Original magnification ×275. *Red signals* indicate mature DC

mature DCs expressing CD83 can be visualized in nodules (Fig. 6.5A). However, some mature DCs expressing CD83 were detected in the adjacent cirrhotic nodules as well (Fig. 6.5B). Although other markers of mature DCs have not been checked in this model, several other investigators have shown the absence of or very few mature DCs in cancer microenvironments. Immature DCs, especially, have been localized in the tumor tissues in some malignancies. In several tumors, a relationship has been found between the frequency of DCs and the tumor prognosis. However, two studies found no relationship between the tumor prognosis and the frequency of infiltrated DCs.

These studies represent the pioneering investigations into the implications of tumor-infiltrating DCs in malignancies. However, several points deserve serious consideration when undertaking studies on tumors of a similar nature. None of these studies was a randomized controlled study, and in most of the investigations there were no proper controls. Furthermore, the tumor tissues were collected from patients with tumors of different stages, and different monoclonal antibodies were used to define DCs. The criteria for determining prognosis were also not well described. Despite the methodological and technical limitations of these studies, a picture of the role of tissue DCs in tumors is emerging.

Table 6.2. Analysis of dendritic cells in tumors

What has been done	What needs to be done
1. Localization of DCs in tumors	Localization of different subsets of DCs in different clinical states of tumors
2. Localization of DCs in established tumors	Localization of DCs in precancerous and cancerous tissues of tumors of the same organ
3. Localization of tumors by various markers	Using standardized markers to identify DCs
4. Localization of bulk population of DCs	Localization of different subtypes of DCs
5. Information regarding functions of tumor-infiltrating DCs	Functional study of tumor-infiltrating DCs

Table 6.2 lists some experiments that have been performed and some that need to be performed to evaluate the clinical implications of the immunohistochemical localization of DCs in tumors.

In most studies, DCs have not been characterized in both precancerous and cancerous tissues of the same organs. Thus, it is hard to assess whether DCs played any role in the initiation of tumorigenesis or whether the nature of the DCs in the tumors reflected the effect of their prolonged exposure to the tumors.

Moreover, there are various subsets of DCs in situ with different types of functional capabilities. Some DCs induce immunity, and others cause tolerance. Although increased frequencies of DCs have been shown to be related to a better prognosis, it is necessary to evaluate what types of DC, immunogenic or tolerogenic, were localized in these studies.

The functions of tumor-infiltrating DCs should be studied in more detail. A functional study should evaluate not only nonspecific functions of DCs, but also their antigen-handling capacity. It is true that these types of studies are extremely hard to conduct in human malignancies, but these limitations must be overcome to take DCs from the lab bench to the bedside.

Implications of Tumor-Infiltrating DCs in Cancer Tissues

Understanding the clinical significance of tumor-infiltrating DCs in tumors is important. DCs in the tumor tissues may take up TAAs and shuttle them to the lymph nodes for the induction of TAA-specific immunity. Although this scenario seems to be too simplistic, experimental evidence either in favor or against it is lacking. Indeed, the presence of increased numbers of immature DCs makes cancer tissues a suitable site for the capture of TAAs. If these DCs capture TAAs, the following considerations are important regarding the function of cancer-infiltrating DCs in cancer tissues.

1. How are these DCs mobilized from blood and what types of signals are required for their mobilization?
2. What is the expression of TLRs and similar receptors on tumor-infiltrating DCs? What is the capacity of these DCs to recognize Ags, especially TAAs?

3. The functional capacity of the Ag-capturing apparatus, such as the capacity to capture TAAs by macropinocytosis, phagocytosis, and receptor-mediated endocytosis of tumor-infiltrating DCs, needs to be defined.
4. The migratory capacity of tumor-infiltrating DCs should be analyzed.
5. The capacity of tumor-infiltrating DCs to undergo maturation and activation following Ag uptake and processing needs to be determined.
6. The ability of tumor-infiltrating DCs to stimulate T cells should be examined.

Cancer-infiltrating DCs may have functional capacities like those of tissue-derived immature DCs. However, if it were found that these DCs are incapable of acting like immature DCs, the important point would to identify the cellular mechanism underlying their dysfunction. For example, tumor-infiltrating DCs in some tumors may have a potent capacity to capture TAAs but may be unable to undergo maturation in the cancer microenvironment. However, in some other cancers, the DCs might not be able to recognize TAAs, although they can undergo maturation in that cancer microenvironment. If the functioning of cancer-infiltrating DCs can be studied in precancerous tissues, more insights will be developed regarding the role of DCs in the initiation of tumorigenesis. This knowledge is also important for the development of DC-based therapies for cancer patients. Until the nature of the defects of DCs in tumor patients is well understood, it will not be possible to determine how to remedy the particular defect involved in a specific tumor. At this time, mature or activated DCs are used for DC-based therapy in patients with tumors, but now is the time to start developing DC-based therapies based on a specific defect of a particular DC function.

DCs with immature phenotype have been detected in tumor tissues. The functional implications of these DCs are outlined in Fig. 6.6. Although there is no scientific data on the factors affecting the localization of mature DCs in tumor tissues, the presence of mature DCs in the vicinity of cancer nodules and their absence in cancer tissues provide indirect evidence that the cancer microenvironment may be hostile to the induction of maturation of DCs in situ. In addition, some in vitro studies have documented that cancer-derived factors block the maturation of DCs. Our present understanding indicates that mature DCs are formed in the lymphoid tissues, not in the peripheral tissues. Although mature DCs have been detected in the peripheral tissues by their expression of phenotypic characteristics, the functions of these DCs have not been studied in detail. It is unknown whether these DCs have already captured Ags and undergone maturation as a result or whether there is an Ag-independent pathway of DC maturation under the influence of local cytokines. It is not impossible that mature DCs in the tissue represent a defective population of DCs that have captured Ags but were unable to move to the lymph nodes because of the ineffective expression of chemokines or their receptors. Whatever the mechanism of formation of mature DCs in cancer tissues might be, it is important to know their functions. If these DCs have not matured in an Ag-dependent manner, they may be source of several cytokines in vivo. TAA-specific CTLs and other lymphocytes migrate to the cancer tissues, although they are formed in the lymphoid tissues. These activated lymphocytes are assigned to kill TAA-expressing tumor cells. However, they may also become apoptotic if certain cytokines are not present in the cancer microenvironment. DCs matured in vitro are a potent source of various cytokines and mediators. Mature DCs in the cancer nodules may be a source of such molecules for the survival and func-

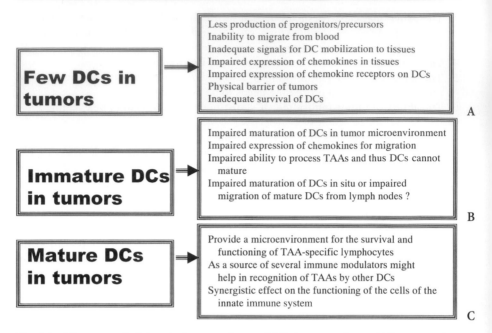

Few DCs in tumors → Less production of progenitors/precursors
Inability to migrate from blood
Inadequate signals for DC mobilization to tissues
Impaired expression of chemokines in tissues
Impaired expression of chemokine receptors on DCs
Physical barrier of tumors
Inadequate survival of DCs

A

Immature DCs in tumors → Impaired maturation of DCs in tumor microenvironment
Impaired expression of chemokines for migration
Impaired ability to process TAAs and thus DCs cannot mature
Impaired maturation of DCs in situ or impaired migration of mature DCs from lymph nodes ?

B

Mature DCs in tumors → Provide a microenvironment for the survival and functioning of TAA-specific lymphocytes
As a source of several immune modulators might help in recognition of TAAs by other DCs
Synergistic effect on the functioning of the cells of the innate immune system

C

Fig. 6.6. **A** Factors underlying the low prevalence of DCs in tumor tissues. **B** Factors underlying the localization of immature DCs in tumors. **C** Mature DCs might induce antitumor immunity

tioning of activated lymphocytes. A lack of mature DCs may thus make the activated lymphocytes more prone to be killed or to undergo apoptosis in vivo.

In certain cancers, such as nasopharyngeal cancer, laryngeal cancer, cervical cancer, esophageal cancer, gastric cancer, lung cancer, and prostate cancers, studies carried out during the last 13 years have shown infiltration of DCs to be related to a positive cancer prognosis, but different investigators used different markers to identify DCs. These results may not be reproducible, because it is not understandable why more DCs in cancer tissues might be associated with a better prognosis. The presence of more DCs may simply reflect a less hostile tumor microenvironment. Thus, a properly controlled study is needed to confirm these results.

Peripheral Blood DCs in Cancer Patients

Although tissue DCs have been characterized in patients with several types of cancer, it is not possible to collect tissue DCs from cancer patients for serial studies. Also, it is not possible to study the phenotypes, functions, and subtypes of tumor-infiltrating DCs, especially in human tumors. Moreover, it is not feasible to study the prognosis of DC-based therapy by analyzing tumor-infiltrating DCs because it is impossible to collect several tissue samples from cancer patients. One way to overcome these problems is to use blood-derived DCs for functional studies. However, it is first necessary to show whether there is any relationship between tumor-infiltrating DCs and blood

DCs in specific tumors. To address this issue, investigators have enriched DCs from the peripheral blood and tumor tissues of patients with tumors. A study on HCC has shown that DCs from these patients had impaired allostimulatory capacity, defective maturation, lower expression of costimulatory molecules such as CD86, and decreased capacity to produce IL-12, a key cytokine required for antitumor immunity. Subsequently, it was confirmed that there were almost no CD83-positive mature DCs in the cancer nodules from these patients, although HLA DR- and S100⁺-positive DCs were detected. It was not possible to isolate DCs from cancer nodules from HCC patients for functional studies. However, it would be important to localize DCs from tumor tissues and to study the functioning of peripheral blood DCs from the same patients to develop more clinically useful insights.

Immunotherapy for Tumors Using Dendritic Cells

Basic Principles and Design of DC-Based Therapies for Tumors

The purpose of tumor immunotherapy is to activate the body's own immune system to fight an existing tumor. This procedure is also called tumor vaccination, but it is much more complex than the vaccination of healthy individuals. The existence of a tumor means that the body's own immune system has been proven to be incapable of inducing a proper antitumor immunity. A tumor may be compared with a massive infection in that there is a huge quantity of cells growing unrestrictedly in many sites of the body. More importantly, when an overt tumor is diagnosed, it has altered the immune system via exhaustion, ignorance, tolerization, or inhibition of antigen-specific cells. Two factors may account for defective antitumor immunity in patients with overt tumors. First, TAAs are usually masked or sequestered inside of the tumor cells, and very few of these Ags may be available on the surface of tumors for recognition by DCs. Moreover, the progressive development of the tumors alters the immune modulatory capacity of the host considerably. To make the matters even worse, a growing tumor creates a local microenvironment, which hampers antigen presentation and elicits the effector function of DCs. Moreover, because of genetic instability, a progressive tumor becomes clonally diverse, which further diminishes the chances that the immune system can recognize and destroy every single tumor clone. In light of these realities, conventional antitumor therapies are not expected to bring about a complete cure. Rather, relapses will occur even from minimal residual disease. A model immune therapy would be able to scan for all tumor cells in every part of the body. Moreover, after their discovery, these tumor cells must be recognized and destroyed without harming the normal tissues surrounding the tumor cells. The current protocols of antitumor chemotherapy and surgical therapy perform none of these functions and thus fail to cure tumors completely. Moreover, immune therapies using activated lymphocytes, killer lymphocytes, and cytokines also fall short. Although most of these therapies are capable of killing tumor cells in vivo, none is able to scan the whole body for tumor cells. Investigations on DCs suggest that full curative therapies for tumors could be achieved by using DCs because these cells are able both to recognize TAAs and induce TAA-specific immunity. Moreover, DCs are capable of scanning the whole body for the presence of residual tumor cells. Most importantly, when residual tumor cells are detected, DCs can induce an antitumor immunity to kill the tumor cells. The stage is now set for successful DC-based immunotherapy for tumors. During the last 10 years, several studies have been conducted in murine experimental tumor models to develop insight into the nature of tumor–DC interactions in vivo and in vitro. At the same time, some clinical trials using DC-based therapy to treat human tumor patients have been undertaken. Understanding the cellular and molecular mechanisms of a DC-based therapy will allow the development of more potent and, finally, perfect DC-based antitumor therapies for tumor-bearing hosts.

To develop a proper immune therapy for tumor patients using DCs, it is important to understand the nature of DCs in tumor-bearing patients. As described in previous chapters, the causes underlying the incapability of DCs to eradicate tumors may be multiple. The following are some potential explanations.

1. DCs may not be able to reach the tumor to take up TAAs. Human papilloma virus-transformed keratinocyte cell lines and HIV inhibit DC migration. The tumor capsule may also act as a barrier blocking DC migration to tumors.

2. Tumors may protect themselves from specific immune reactions via the production of factors that prevent DCs from migrating from the tumor to the regional lymph nodes.

3. DCs may not recognize the tumors as "dangerous" and "nonself."

4. By producing immunosuppressive factors, tumors may compromise the functioning of DCs and make them unable to induce antitumor immunity. DCs in prostate cancer tissues are minimally activated. DCs in basal cell carcinomas fail to express costimulatory molecules such as CD80 or CD86. In colorectal cancers, DCs do not express CD80 or CD86. IL-10 also negatively regulates the functioning of DCs. In a growing melanoma, DCs reside in a microenvironment with IL-10, but in a regressing melanoma, IL-10 cannot be detected near DCs. Other tumor-derived factors such as transforming growth factor (TGF)-β, vascular endothelial growth factor, and prostaglandins may negatively regulate the functioning of DCs.

5. Many drugs that are used for cancer therapy may also downregulate DC functioning. Steroids, which are a component of many chemotherapeutic regimens, are powerful inhibitors of the development and differentiation of DCs. Steroids also impair the antigen-presenting capacity of DCs. Anticancer drugs may also induce IL-10 and regulatory T cells, which downregulate the functioning of DCs.

In summary, inhibition of normal DC physiology by the tumor itself, by medication, or by deliberate exposure to external immune-compromising factors might allow tumor progression. Circumstantial evidence supports the idea that tumors can employ numerous means to inhibit the migration, activation, and antigen-presentation function of DCs.

Optimization of DC-Based Therapy for Human Tumors

Introduction

Clinical studies of DC-based immunotherapy were first performed in patients with advanced cancers, and these initial studies reported occasional regressions of

Factors related to DC-based immunotherapy	Variables
A. Types of DCs	Myeloid or plasmacytoid or both
B. Loading with TAAs	Pulsing, transfection, fusion, exosome
C. Dose and frequency	Low dose/high dose; frequencies
D. Route of administration	s.c., i.d., i.v., intranodal, intratumor
E. Migration	Treatment with pulsed DCs with migratory factors
F. Activation/maturation	Treatment with TAA-loaded DCs with activation factors
G. Survival	Manipulation to increase survival in vivo

A

Evaluation of therapeutic responses	
Antitumor immunity	Direct evaluation of TAA-specific
Tumor size	Regression/unchanged/increased
Survival	Increased/unchanged/unaffected
Recurrence	Local/distant recurrence
Side effects	Autoimmunity/local response

B

Fig. 6.7A,B. Effective DC-based therapy for tumors might be developed by selecting proper types of DCs, adequately loading TAAs on DCs, fixing the proper doses of DCs, and optimizing the frequency and route of administration of DCs. The migration of these injected DCs and their ability to activate lymphocytes are also important factors (**A**). The therapeutic evaluation of DC-based therapy should be based on the intensity of the antitumor immunity as well as on the survival of the tumor-bearing hosts (**B**)

metastatic lesions following DC-based therapy. The phase I clinical trials indicated that there were few side effects of repeated injections of autologous DCs in cancer patients. Subsequently, studies of healthy volunteers and patients with tumors provided extremely important information for designing the protocols of DC-based immunotherapy for tumors.

The following factors should be considered when designing DC-based therapy for tumors (Fig. 6.7).

1. Factors concerning the type of DCs that should be used to induce appropriate T-cell responses during DC-based therapy. The sources of the DCs are important in this regard.
2. Factors affecting the loading of TAAs on DCs.
3. Dose, frequency and route of administration of DCs.
4. Factors related to the migration of administered DCs.

Types and Sources of DCs

The purpose of DC-based therapy for tumor-bearing hosts is to induce TAA-specific antitumor immunity. Mature DCs are able to polarize CD4$^+$ T cells toward the Th1 phenotype, which is important for host resistance because these cells produce IFN-γ.

This cytokine also has an anti-angiogenic effect that may influence the survival and metastasis of tumors. Moreover, Th1 cells home better to sites of inflammation and thus can provide better antitumor activity. In addition, Th1 cells may activate DCs better to sustain CD8$^+$ T-cell function, especially in the case of a persistent viral and tumor antigen load.

In addition, mature DCs help to establish memory CTL responses. Moreover, mature DCs are able to aid in the production of protective antibodies by B cells. Mature DCs also play a vital role in the establishment and maintenance of T-cell memory by producing IL-15. The CD8$^+$ T cells produced by the influence of mature DCs can be activated by a low dose of Ags. This is an important factor in tumor settings because only very small amounts of TAAs may be available in situ.

In contrast, immature DCs are mostly ignored by the immune system. Interactions between immature DCs and T cells result in the formation of T regulatory (T^{reg}) cells. These cells can silence the immune system. T^{reg} cells produce IL-10 and act as a negative regulator of the immune response.

DC-based immune therapy began by using monocyte-derived DCs. These offer the advantages of high yield, purity, and feasibility, especially when leukapheresis is used to collect the starting monocytes. These DCs can also be successfully cryopreserved, even after loading with antigens.

DCs derived from CD34$^+$ HPCs have also been used for DC-based therapy. A clinical study with CD34-derived DCs resulted in short-term immunity and clinical efficacy. These DCs comprise a mixture of two subsets of DCs: Langerhans cells or epidermal DCs and monocyte-derived or interstitial DCs. These two DC subsets differ in the markers present and some functions. For example, Langerhans cells are ineffective at stimulating B-cell development directly, a function that may require the expression of B-cell activating factor belonging to the tumor necrosis factor (TNF) family (BAFF) on monocyte-derived DCs. CD34-derived DCs may be better at eliciting CTLs.

Recently, a DC subset called plasmacytoid DCs has been characterized. These cells can be collected from the peripheral blood. They are lineage$^-$, CD4$^+$, HLA DR$^+$, CD123$^+$, CD11c$^-$. The most striking difference between plasmacytoid DCs and monocyte-derived DCs may be their migratory capacity. Plasmacytoid DCs respond to IL-3 and express CD62L or L-selectin; thus, they can home directly to T-cell areas via high endothelial venules. Monocyte-derived DCs are produced by culturing monocytes with GM-CSF and IL-4; they lack CD62L and probably must go to the tissues and traverse the afferent lymphatics before accessing the T-cell areas of the lymphoid tissues. The expression of TLRs is also different on these two DC populations. Plasmacytoid cells express TLR7 and TLR9, and monocyte-derived DCs express TLR2 and TLR4. Monocyte-derived DCs can produce high amounts of IL-12 upon stimulation with CD40L, whereas plasmacytoid DCs produce large amounts of IFN-α with certain enveloped viruses. However, IFN-α produced by plasmacytoid DCs can induce the maturation and activation of monocyte-derived DCs and NK cells. Mature monocyte-derived and plasmacytoid-derived DCs have the potential to induce either Th1$^+$ or Th2$^+$ CD4 T-cell responses. To date, no study including clinical trials of tumor therapies using plasmacytoid DCs or a mixture of plasmacytoid and monocyte-derived DCs has been done.

Loading of DCs with TAAs

DCs are not expected to take up TAAs in vivo from cancer tissues; accordingly, DCs should be loaded with TAAs or their peptides during DC-based immunotherapy. Although loading of DCs in vitro with peptides from TAAs would be ideal, there are significant limitations in the use of peptides as the source of TAAs. The following are methods used to load DCs with TAAs.

Transfection with Tumor-Derived RNA. Transfection of DCs with RNA derived from tumor tissues could lead to the expression of a wide variety of tumor peptides on DCs. The RNA could be used directly or after amplification from small amounts of starting material. Only a few tumor cells in a biopsy would be needed in most instances. These RNA approaches have the potential to elicit immune responses to proteins uniquely expressed in a patient's tumor. However, some of the proteins produced from the transfected total RNA may have immune inhibitory capacity in vivo.

Transfection Using Viral Vectors. Adenoviral vectors encoding the genes of target proteins can be efficiently transfected into immature DCs. These transfected DCs have been shown to undergo maturation with the standard stimuli and to carry out normal functions such as IL-12 production, antigen presentation to CD8$^+$ T cells, and the induction of antitumor immunity in mice.

This transfection can also be done using poxvirus vectors. However, the infection is abortive, with only early viral gene products being expressed. Furthermore, when immature DCs are infected, infection is followed by overt cytotoxicity. Nevertheless, efficient presentation of the recombinant gene is observed in culture, possibly through cross-presentation of dying infected DCs by other noninfected DCs.

Several other virus vectors such as retroviruses, lentiviruses, and influenza virus can be used to transfect DCs.

The viral vectors mentioned above are used to infect DCs ex vivo. Some viral envelopes may also prove useful to directly and selectively target DCs in vivo. The HIV-1 envelope may target DCs via a lectin called DC-specific ICAM-3-grabbing nonintegrin (DC-SIGN). The lymphocytic choriomeningitis virus (LCMV) targets mouse DCs via α-dystroglycan and the dengue virus targets human LCs and monocyte derived DCs. In summary, some viral envelopes provide potential DC-targeting strategies. This approach will be highly useful when manipulation of DCs is done in vivo.

Receptor-Mediated Uptake of Proteins by DCs. DCs are equipped with several Ag-internalization machineries. These include macropinocytosis, where specific aquaporins appear to be essential for the influx and efflux of fluid. In phagocytosis, several different receptors contribute to the uptake of cells. Adsorptive uptake is mediated via clathrin-coated vesicles, such as the mannose receptor-mediated uptake of certain glycoproteins (gps). Uptake by fluid-phase pinocytosis and phagocytosis usually ceases upon full maturation of the DCs, but adsorptive pinocytosis via clathrin-coated vesicles can persist.

One DC receptor, DEC-205, greatly enhances the efficiency of MHC class II-mediated presentation after the adsorptive uptake step. DEC-205 is unique because it does not recycle through peripheral endosomes, as is typical for most adsorptive receptors. Instead, the cytosolic domain is able to move the receptor more deeply into the cell through MHC II late endosomes or lysosomes. This unusual traffic pattern is associated with a 10- to 100-fold increase in the presentation of ligands compared with the classical macrophage mannose receptor, which recycles through peripheral endosomes.

Several pathways target the MHC class I compartments of DCs, which is remarkable because in most cells MHC I molecules are loaded from newly synthesized proteins. For some of these "exogenous" pathways to MHC class I, specific receptors are known, such as the Fcγ receptor for immune complexes. Heat shock proteins (hsp), particularly hsp70, can deliver peptides to MHC class I in vivo. Heat shock proteins are therefore being considered as adjuvants for peptide delivery to DCs and even for modifying other aspects of DC function such as maturation. As in the case of viral vectors, the ex vivo use of heat shock proteins allows control of the DC targeting step as well as of DC maturation.

Loading of Dead or Dying Tumor Cells or Cell Lines. This pathway allows DCs to phagocytose tumor cells or their fragments. Cross-presentation by DCs was first described with viral peptides from apoptotic, infected cells. It is now evident that tumor-associated peptides can also be presented, and from just one to two dead cells per DC. Both apoptotic and necrotic types of cell death can be followed by cross-presentation. In some instances, necrotic cells also mature the DCs and release gp96.

However, there are some limitations to the use of tumor cells as the source of antigens. Dead cells loaded with self-peptides can lead to autoimmunity. It is now evident that presentation of dying cells by DCs induces tolerance to self-peptides. It has been proposed, however, that most patients are already tolerant to many of the self-peptides that DCs are able to process.

The major potential of the use of tumor cells as the source of antigens is that it allows DCs to be charged with a wide array of tumor peptides and with both MHC class I and class II molecules.

Fusion Between DCs and Tumor Cells. Another strategy for delivering several tumor antigens to DCs is to fuse the two cell types, creating heterokaryons. Fused mixtures of tumor cells and DCs enhance resistance to mouse mammary tumors, human ovarian cancer, HCC, and advanced renal cancer. Although these results are encouraging, they are puzzling as well because heterokaryons between different cell types, here DCs and tumor cells, are normally unstable.

Exosomes. Exosomes are small, membrane-bound vesicles that are either released from tumor cells or presented by DCs. They may also be released by DCs that have processed tumor cells. Exosomes contain MHC class I and II products, costimulatory molecules such as CD86, and other cell-derived products such as heat shock proteins. However, it may not be feasible to obtain the large amounts of tumor cells needed for this approach from most patients. However, exosomes could be developed into a standard form of tumor antigen, which would be captured and presented by DCs in vivo or by ex vivo derived DCs. This will require methods to charge the exosomes with tumor-derived antigenic peptides and to ensure the maturation of DCs within the cancer-bearing patient.

Dose, Frequency, and Route of Administration of DCs

The dose of DCs is important in the context of DC-based antitumor immunotherapy. There is little information regarding the effect of DC dose on the subsequent antitumor immune response in vivo. Studies in vitro have shown that a low dose of DCs, like a low dose of antigens, can polarize T cells toward the Th2 pathway. However, the dose of injected DCs should not be too large because that may hinder their access to the lymphatics.

The frequency of injection of DCs is also an important factor. After injection, DCs systematically induce a series of cellular events, the final product being Ag-specific CTLs. These CTLs are located in the lymphoid tissues but eventually migrate to the tissue of localization of tumors. A rapid injection schedule may result in the DCs being killed by the CTLs, because the injected DCs would express tumor Ags. This makes them an easy target for destruction by Ag-specific CTLs.

The immunogenicity of DCs after different routes of administration in humans also needs to be compared. Some data suggest that the subcutaneous and intradermal routes lead to greater nodal migration compared with the intravenous route of administration. The first two injection protocols also result in improved Th1 polarization. Recently, DCs have been injected directly into the lymph nodes with the intent to cause direct interaction with T cells. However, the antitumor effect of intranodal administration of DCs has not been evaluated in clinical trials.

A new approach is to inject DCs directly into the tumor. This may enhance the afferent limb of immunity in vivo. A portion of the tumor was necrotized by alcohol, a necrotizing agent, and then, after 48 hours, bone marrow-derived, immature DCs were injected. The purpose was to pulse immature DCs in vivo with all available TAAs and to provide certain maturation signals, which may come from the necrotizing tissues. Administration of DCs in this manner resulted in increased survival and decreased tumor size in tumor-bearing mice. Seventy-two hours after administration of immature DCs, mature DCs expressing CD11c and CD86 were detected in the tumor nodules (Fig. 6.8A). These injected DCs in the tumors might undergo maturation in the tumor microenvironment or they may mature in the secondary lymphoid organs, because some of the labeled immature DCs were localized in the spleen 48 h after their injection into the tumor nodules (Fig. 6.8B). This approach has the advantage of loading DCs with all available TAAs in vivo. However, the effect of tumor microenvironments on the Ag-capturing capacity of immature DCs deserves further study.

Migration of Injected DCs During Immunotherapy

After internalization and processing of Ags, the migration of DCs to the draining lymph node and their longevity upon reaching the node are important factors affecting the efficacy of DC-based therapy. In mice, treatment of DCs with CD40L enhances their migration from the tissues to the lymph nodes. However, only a very small number of the injected DCs could be traced in the draining lymph node (10% or less). The expression of CCR7 on DCs is required for effective migration. The chemokines MIP-3β and SLC, which are made by the lymphatics, should also be expressed for the efficient migration of DCs.

It is also important to evaluate the therapeutic potential of DC-based therapies. I suggest some generalized evaluation criteria in Fig. 6.7B. However, criteria appropriate for determining complete responders and partial responders would depend on the study population and the nature of the tumor.

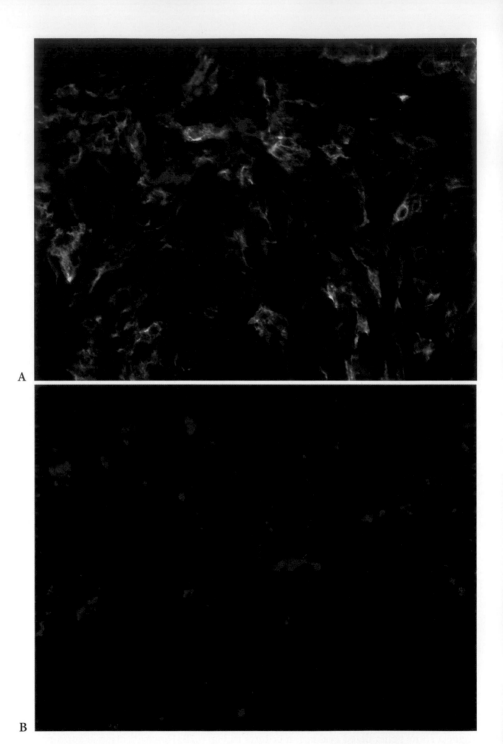

Fig. 6.8A,B. Bone marrow-derived immature DCs were injected into cancer nodules, 48 h after necrotizing a part of experimental colon cancer tissues with 100% ethanol, a necrotizing agent. Although mature DCs co-expressing CD11c and CD86 were not seen in untreated cancer nodules, this procedure caused localization of mature DCs in cancer nodules. Mature DC is shown by *Yellow signals* (**A**). The localization of bone marrow-derived immature DCs in the spleen 72 h after their administration into the cancer nodules (**B**) indicated that some of the DCs migrated to the spleen. DCs were labeled with PKH 26 to trace their migration. Original magnification ×450. PKH-26 labelled DC was shown as *red*

DC-Based Immune Therapy in Human Tumors

From several studies in vitro it has become apparent that tumors might be ignored by DCs, they might suppress DC function, or they might be presented with immature DCs that induce T^{reg} cells. Thus, there is a need to amplify the afferent limb of the immune system and to bypass the potential defects in the presentation of TAAs in vivo. This can be achieved by loading DCs with TAAs in vitro. The initial DC studies were designed to demonstrate the feasibility, that is, lack of acute toxicity and responses to MHC class I-restricted tumor peptides, of DC-based immune therapy. Many of the first human protocols were designed to use DCs that were probably immature, which may be suboptimal in many respects. Despite these problems, and even though basic information such as optimal cell dose and route of injection are unknown, antigen-bearing DCs enhanced immunity in humans and induced clinical regression in some patients with advanced cancer. Initially, short-term vaccinations were carried out over a period of a few months. Studies with a longer follow-up or with revaccination strategies are underway to test the potential of antigen-bearing DCs to stabilize metastatic disease or even induce complete remission.

Melanoma

Melanoma is the best-studied tumor from an immunologic perspective. In contrast to other tumors where little is known regarding TAAs, several melanoma antigens have been defined. Some of these antigens are also expressed in normal tissues; therefore, the possibility of tolerance to these antigens exists. Several DC-based studies have been carried out in patients with stage IV melanoma. When DCs were pulsed with melanoma peptides, including MAGE-3, tyrosinase, gp100, and Melan A/MART1, immune responses to the peptides were detectable, indicating that tolerance to these antigens was partial. However, their capacity to increase T cell numbers and to kill melanoma targets needs to be assessed. In one clinical trial in which 18 stage IV melanoma patients were injected subcutaneously with CD34-derived DCs pulsed with tumor peptides, the DCs induced antigen-specific T cells. Vitiligo flared markedly in some patients, although they had a history of vitiligo attack before the administration of DC-based therapy. The preliminary data suggest a correlation between immune responses and early clinical outcome. The clinical trials in melanoma patients not only indicate a role for DC-based therapy in these patients, but melanoma may also be used as a disease model for optimizing conditions for more robust immune responses to achieve further clinical efficacy.

Prostate Cancer

In most published studies, tissue-specific self-antigens such as prostate-specific Ag (PSA) have been targeted by DC-based therapies, using either blood DCs or monocyte-derived DCs. The levels of serum PSA, which reflects the tumor burden, were reduced in about 25% of patients. In two studies, injection of blood-derived DCs pulsed with Ag fusion protein led to a greater than 50% reduction in serum PSA in some patients. In these studies, the evidence for immunogenicity of DCs was based on antigen-specific proliferative responses after vaccination. Prostate cancer offers two key challenges for research in DC therapy: the availability of serum markers to follow tumor-cell burden and defined prostate-restricted antigens and carcinoma lines to monitor the T-cell immune response.

Lymphoma and Myeloma

The target selected in published studies for both of these tumors is a tumor-specific antigen, the idiotype of the monoclonal Ig expressed as a surface receptor or secreted by the tumor. In some studies, patients also received soluble antigen, which complicated the evaluation of the response. Occasional tumor regressions were observed in some patients with lymphoma. Both low-grade, non-Hodgkin's lymphoma and myeloma respond to, but are not cured by, standard chemotherapy and may therefore be amenable to vaccination in the setting of minimal residual disease.

Virus-Associated Malignancies

In virus-associated malignancies, virus-derived antigens that are foreign to the immune system serve as attractive targets for immune therapy. However, one major problem would be chronic viral infection, when the viral antigens behave like self-antigens. Examples of such viruses and associated malignancies include hepatitis C virus and HCC, human papillomavirus and cervical cancer, Epstein-Barr virus (EBV), and lymphoma or nasopharyngeal cancer. Vaccination approaches have begun to target cervical cancer caused by human papillomaviruses, but the immunity induced with the current non-DC adjuvant appears weak. In some virus-related malignancies, mucosal immunization may be valuable. DCs can be visualized beneath the antigen-transporting epithelium of mucosa-associated lymphoid tissues. The CCR6 chemokine receptor, initially studied in the setting of epidermal DCs, now appears to be important for the capacity of DCs to initiate immunity to antigens deposited in mucosal sites.

Renal Cancer

Renal cancer is resistant to chemotherapy but can occasionally respond to cytokines such as IL-2. DCs have been charged with crude lysates of autologous tumors, but one study used fusions of allogenic DCs and patient-derived renal cancer cells. Of 17 patients, 6 underwent striking regressions of their cancers. The underlying mechanisms are not yet clear, but the allogenic DCs may have induced IL-2 and, in turn, NK cells, to which renal carcinoma cells are sensitive.

Other Tumors

Immunotherapy directed against other tumors falls broadly into two categories: one is to target defined antigens such as overexpressed self-antigens (Her2/neu, CEA, muc-1) and mutant oncoproteins (bcr-abl, p53, mutant ras) and another is to use crude antigenic preparations derived from autologous tumor lysates, peptides eluted with acid from cells, tumor-derived RNA, or heat shock proteins. Injection of tumor lysate-pulsed DCs led to marked tumor regression in a child with metastatic fibrosarcoma.

Future of DC-Based Therapy in Human Tumors

Cautions and Limitations

From the discussion so far, it is evident that DCs are not only important but play a critical role in the generation of tumor immunity in vivo. Based on data on the therapeutic efficacy of DC-based therapy in murine experimental tumors, DC-based therapy has been begun in human tumor patients around the world. The published results of these clinical trials are also encouraging, at least initially, as these DC-based therapies have mainly been attempted in patients with advanced cancers.

However, some realities require serious cautions regarding these therapies. If DCs are so important for cancer immunity, DC-derived cancers should not exist because the tumor cells should be able to efficiently present endogenously produced tumor Ags. Although neoplasms of DCs are rare, cancers of DC origin have nevertheless been described. Langerhans cell histocytosis and interdigital dendritic cell sarcoma are two major cancers of DCs. These cancer cells express CD83. Recently, plasmacytoid DCs have been found to be malignantly transformed into a special form of lymphoma.

Several explanations for these observations are possible. The rarity of DC cancer may point to high antigenicity, which normally would not allow uncontrolled tumor growth because of effective autopresentation. On the other hand, the proven existence of neoplastic diseases originating from transformed DCs further points to the fact that, although DCs are very powerful APCs, the mere presence of even large amounts of antigen-bearing DCs alone is not necessarily sufficient to induce tumor immunity. Another possibility is that the DCs forming the basis of malignant disease are in an immature stage and thus induce tolerance rather than immunity against themselves, as the induction of tolerance has been shown to be a function of immature DCs.

Hopes and Prospects

It is important to evaluate what we know about tumors and to propose problems that we should address for the development of DC-based immunotherapy for tumors. Tumor immunology lies at the intersection of two large, complex, and somewhat inbred disciplines: tumor research and immunology. Therefore, tumor immunology is best thought as of two fields: one that uses tumors as a model system in which to test immunological principles, and another that uses immunology as a tool for understanding and treating tumors. DCs, as the most professional APCs, as the accessory cells of the immune system, and as the regulators of immune responses, are part of this conjoined field. The ultimate target of studies of DCs in tumors is to learn how basic concepts can be integrated, synthesized, and applied to real problems of human tumors. From this point of view, DC research remains in its infancy. Many of the roles of DCs in tumor immunology have been investigated in experiments in murine cancer models. Success is measured by the extent to which the basic concepts are tested and refined and not by their impact on human cancers. In fact, there is tremendous bias among scientists and clinicians that this is the ultimate result. However, tumors in humans are in no way comparable to the reproducible, well-defined, cell-based animal models. Moreover, the extensive complexity of DC lineage is very hard to study properly in humans. Tumor antigens in humans are highly variable, and the optimum methodology for loading them is also very hard to understand. Considerations that may be important for DC-based therapy are listed in Fig. 6.7. With all these limitations, the use of DC-based therapies for human tumors has begun, and some of these therapies have shown promising outcomes. Methods have been developed to enrich huge numbers of DCs in vitro. More and more TAAs are being characterized. We are learning how DCs can be loaded with TAAs in vitro by several methods and gaining information regarding the dose, duration, and route of administration of DCs. However, we are still not sure whether DC-based vaccines can prevent tumors in humans or how such vaccines should be administered. It is still unknown whether DCs have any role in the initiation or progression of human cancers. It is not even clear whether the administration of DCs might exacerbate cancer in some patients. DC-based therapy has usually been attempted in patients with advanced cancer, and it has not been possible to properly follow up these patients. This therapy does not induce autoimmunity in patients with advanced cancer, but the immune system of these patients has already failed. Would autoimmunity be induced by DC-based therapy in young immune-competent patients? On the other hand, we should look for defects in the different limbs of DC functioning in cancers by evaluating whether the defect lies in the mobilization, Ag recognition, Ag capture, Ag processing, migration, or Ag presentation of DCs in different cancers.

These precautions are not intended to discourage the development of DC-based immune therapy, but to offer some historical perspective . Many prospective immune therapies have not stood the test of time, although most inspired initial optimism.

Theoretically, DCs are capable of scanning the whole body for the presence of tumor cells in normal conditions, in precancerous conditions, and even after the development of overt cancers. They can induce tumor-specific immunity in vivo. They are also able to produce groups of fighters known as memory cells for future attacks. None of these activities can be performed by any existing antitumor therapy. We need to explore the nature of tumors with a case-by-case perspective and understand the different types of DCs.

Recommended Readings

Byrne SC, Hallyday GM (2002) Dendritic cells: making progress with tumor regression. Immunol Cell Biol 80:520–530

Brossart P, Wirths S, Brugger W, et al. (2001) Dendritic cells in cancer vaccines. Exp Hematol 29:1247–1255

Dallal RM, Lotze MT (2000) The dendritic cell and human cancer vaccines. Curr Opin Immunol 12:583–588

Fong L, Engleman EG (2002) Dendritic cells in cancer immunotherapy. Annu Rev Immunol 18:245–273

Gunzer M, Janich S, Varga G, et al. (2001) Dendritic cells and tumor immunity. Semin Immunol 13:291–302

Hart DN (1997) Dendritic Cells: unique leukocyte populations which control the primary immune respone. Blood 90:3245–3287

Matsue H, Kusuhara M, Matsue K, et al. (2002) Dendritic cell-based immunoregulatory strategies. Int Arch Allergy Immunol 127:251–258

Nestle FO (2002) Dendritic cell vaccination for cancer therapy. Oncogene 19:6673–6679

Onji M, Akbar SMF, Horiike N (2001) Dendritic cell-based immunotherapy for hepatocellular carcinoma. J Gastroenterol 36:794–797

Schuler G, Schuler-Thurner B, Steinman RM (2003) The use of dendritic cells in cancer immunotherapy. Curr Opin Immunol 15:138–147

Sprinzi GM, Kacani L, Schrott-Fischer A, et al. (2001) Dendritic cell vaccines for cancer therapy. Cancer Treat Rev 27:247–255

Steinman RM, Dhodapkar M (2001) Active immunization against cancer with dendritic cells: the near future. Int J Cancer 94:459–473

Steinman RM, Pope M (2002) Exploiting dendritic cells to improve vaccine therapy. J Clin Invest 109:1519–1526

Tatsumi T, Storkins WJ (2002) Dendritic cell-based vaccines and therapies for cancers. Expert Opin Biol Ther 2:919–928

7. Dendritic Cells in Transplantation

Involvement of Dendritic Cells During Transplantation

Tremendous developments in surgical procedures, application of anesthetics, and technical understanding of the preservation of organs in transplantation have occurred during the last two to three decades, bringing about a silent revolution in organ transplantation. Indeed, there are several diseases for which transplantation has become the only choice to save the life of a patient. From a surgical point of view, the transplantation operation is usually successful; however, the life-long management of transplantation patients is very difficult. The acute and chronic rejection of the transplanted organs are major problems following transplantation. In most cases, the patients are given immunosuppressive drugs for the rest of their lives, which greatly compromises the quality of life. Two approaches might solve these problems. The first would be to generate artificial organs and to optimize their clinical use. This would definitely revolutionize organ transplantation, but it is unlikely to be realized in the near future. The second approach would be to develop insights into the causes underlying the rejection of allografts and to develop remedies to prevent that rejection. Donor organs that are transplanted into an allogenic recipient contain several types of cells, including parenchymal cells, nonparenchymal cells (endothelial cells, fibroblasts, vascular cells, and specialized cells of the specific transplanted organ), and various types of cells of the immune system. All types of cells from the donor may play a role in the rejection of transplanted organs because all of them have allogenic major histocompatibility complex (MHC) antigens. However, the cells of the immune system would be dominant in this regard because some of them express both MHC class II and class I antigens. Moreover, the cells of the immune system are migratory, and those from the donor might undergo maturation and activation in the recipient, providing them with additional ability to induce an alloantigen-specific immune response in the recipient. The role of immunocytes in transplant rejection became evident when it was shown that depletion, deactivation, and suppression of leukocyte populations in donor organs improved the chances of allograft acceptance. To deplete leukocytes in donor organs, researchers developed techniques, such as culturing them in low-temperature and hyperbaric oxygen conditions, during the mid-1970s. In addition, some investigators used an intermediate transplantation approach, in which a donor organ was first transplanted into an intermediate host under severe immune suppressive conditions. This led to severe functional impairment of the leukocytes in the donor organ, which was then retransplanted from the intermediate host into the

131

final recipient. Depletion and functional impairment of leukocyte populations led to increased survival of allografts after transplantation.

These investigations suggested that donor leukocytes are involved in the rejection of allografts, but it remained unclear which types of leukocytes were primarily responsible for rejection. The immune responses that contribute to the rejection of allografts are comparable to the immune reaction that occurs in an allogenic mixed lymphocyte reaction (MLR) or mixed leukocyte culture in vitro. As antigen-presenting dendritic cells (DCs) are the most potent stimulators of allogenic MLRs, a dominant role of DCs in the rejection of allografts was predicted. DCs express very high levels of MHC class II and class I antigens. During allogenic MLRs, DCs present alloantigens to allogenic T cells and induce their proliferation. In addition to their strong capacity to stimulate allogenic MLRs, DCs can act as initiators, propagators, and regulators of the immune response. DCs may become activated as a result of the alteration of the mucosal milieu in the tissue microenvironment after transplantation. DCs are passenger leukocytes and are capable of migrating to the lymphoid tissues for presenting alloantigens and other antigens for the induction of immune responses. In transplantation, the surgical intervention might be the most potent stimulus for the activation and maturation of DCs. These activated DCs would be most likely to migrate to the lymphoid tissues of the recipients, where they can directly activate T cells. They can also release antigens from their MHC groove and thus may indirectly activate T cells. All these activities of the donor DCs would make the rejection of allografts more likely.

On the other hand, DCs not only induce immune responses, they are also potent inducers of immune tolerance. DCs are not a homogenous cell population; rather, there are subtypes of DCs in both human and mouse. Some of these subtypes are committed inducers of immune tolerance. In addition, cytokines and immune modulators can alter the nature of DCs. Under the influence of cytokines, immunogenic DCs can become tolerogenic DCs.

Many studies suggest that DCs might be a foe in the context of transplantation because they induce an immune response and make allograft rejection more likely. However, if donor DCs can be altered to a tolerogenic population, that would definitely increase the chance of acceptance of allografts. In addition, the functions of DCs could be downregulated in vivo by using one of several approaches. However, the use of DCs in transplant patients requires understanding of the nature of DCs and of ways of manipulating them. In this chapter, I discuss DCs both as friends and foes of transplantation.

Dendritic Cells in Allograft Rejection

DCs are foes because they cause allograft rejection after transplantation. More precisely, DCs of the donor are the main culprit in the rejection of allografts. Donor DCs are in the best position to induce an immune response against recipient alloantigens. However, DCs from both the donor and the recipient might constitute a formidable obstacle to allograft acceptance. The cellular and molecular mechanisms of allograft rejection and the activities of DCs cannot be studied in detail in human models of transplantation. However, insights into these mechanisms have been acquired from animal experimentation and by analyzing immunological events in allogenic MLRs. During the initial phase of allogenic MLRs, discrete aggregates of DCs and T cells are formed. Allogenic DCs can directly stimulate purified CD4$^+$ and CD8$^+$ T lymphocytes in allogenic MLRs, resulting in the growth and proliferation of T cells, which leads to the production of T blasts. Once T blasts are formed by DCs, other APCs such as macrophages and B cells can also induce vigorous proliferation of T blasts.

After transplantation, donor DCs migrate to the lymphoid tissue of the recipients, where they induce alloantigen-specific activation of recipient T cells. The surgical procedure of transplantation might provide stimulatory and activation signals for the induction of immune responses. The donor allograft contains several DC populations, such as immature DCs, tolerogenic DCs, DC precursors, and DC progenitors. In vitro, immature DCs are poor activators of allogenic T cells, but the capabilities of different populations of donor DCs to stimulate allogenic T cells of the recipient have not been examined. It is very important to note that the phenotypes and maturational status of DCs in the donor organs may be altered by anesthesia, preservation technique, or surgical manipulations. Liver allografts are well accepted even with an MHC mismatch. Liver harbors considerable numbers of DC progenitors with very special phenotypes and functions. In contrast to immature DCs and DC precursors, liver DC progenitors do not undergo maturation in the presence of known stimulatory signals such as tumor necrosis factor (TNF)-α and interferon (IFN)-γ. This difference might underlie the excellent acceptance of liver allografts even with an MHC mismatch; however, this remains to be confirmed.

What would initiate the migration of DCs in the donor allograft to recipient lymphoid tissues? Chemokines may play a role in this situation. However, parenchymal factors may also be important. Increased expression of ligands for Toll-like receptors (TLRs) in the recipient parenchymal cells might also induce maturation of DCs. The expression of TLRs on donor DCs would also be important in this regard. An involvement of the Toll system is suspected, but not confirmed, in transplant rejection.

T cells can recognize the MHC alloantigens by two distinct pathways: "direct" or "indirect." In the direct pathway of allorecognition, T-cell receptors of alloreactive T cells ligate with the foreign MHC antigens on DCs. The donor DCs then migrate to recipient lymphoid tissues, where recipient T cells are subsequently activated.

In the indirect pathway of allorecognition, T cells recognize allogenic MHC molecules as peptides presented in the context of self-MHC antigens. This recognition system is somewhat similar to that used for the recognition of nominal antigens. DCs of the donor are a source for various antigens. Immature DCs of the donor may have engulfed various apoptotic and necrotic bodies, which may have undergone processing in the donor DCs. These DCs would migrate to the lymphoid tissues of the recipient. In the lymphoid tissues, MHC peptides might be eluted from the peptide-binding grooves of the MHC molecules, and these eluted MHC peptides would be captured by recipient DCs as nominal soluble antigens. After processing the captured antigens, recipient DCs would activate alloantigen-specific T cells, which would lead to the activation and proliferation of T cells. The role of macrophages as a source of eluted MHC molecules is controversial. Although macrophages possess high potentiality to capture apoptotic cells and other dying cells, they probably digest the antigens completely and thus cannot supply the antigen in peptide form to recipient T cells.

Acute and Chronic Rejection

In general, it is thought that acute rejection is the end product of direct allorecognition. Donor DCs as passenger leukocytes are released or they migrate from the allograft to the recipient tissues. The roles of various chemokines and signals in their migration from the donor tissue have not been well explored, but these DCs would be a powerful stimulus for the proliferation of recipient allogenic T cells. In addition, the interaction between DCs and T cells would lead to Th1 polarization and production of various inflammatory cytokines.

Traditionally, it has been assumed that chronic rejection is the result of indirect allorecognition. This is suggested by a largely indolent, but progressive form of allograft injury characterized primarily by persistent, but patchy inflammation of the allograft, fibrointimal hyperplasia of arteries, interstitial fibrosis, and destruction and atrophy of parenchymal elements and organ-associated lymphoid tissue. In contrast to acute rejection, chronic rejection develops over a longer period. Although indirect allorecognition, which allows the recipient's DCs to present donor MHC peptides to autologous T cells, might be one of the main factors underlying the development of chronic rejection, chronic rejection also develops in many cases from inadequately controlled acute rejection and in patients not compliant with immunosuppressive therapy. These observations point to the activation of DCs in situ. Infiltration of the allograft by recipient accessory cells, including macrophages and DCs, is a hallmark of chronic rejection. The inflammatory infiltrates in chronic rejection are often arranged as nodular aggregates, some of which contain a germinal center in secondary lymphoid follicles. The number of recipient DCs in chronically rejecting organs directly correlates with the overall severity of inflammation.

DCs in Tolerance Induction: Therapeutic Implications

DCs of both donor and recipient origin may act as foes, causing acute, as well as chronic, rejection of allografts. Direct allorecognition by donor DCs is thought to induce acute rejection, whereas indirect allorecognition by recipient DCs causes chronic rejection. As the immune response to alloantigens causes the rejection of allografts, it might be possible to reverse the process by manipulating the functioning of DCs. However, DCs have diverse functions, and it is important to understand the DC function that is to be manipulated in order to develop a DC-based therapy for transplantation. The relative contributions of direct and indirect allorecognition have been examined in a murine model of skin graft rejection. In this model, during acute rejection, 90% of the responding T cells responded to directly presented donor MHC peptides, whereas, less than 10% of T cells recognized allopeptides presented indirectly.

Induction of Immune Tolerance by Manipulating DC–T Cell Interactions

The predominant role of the direct pathway provides a rational basis for the manipulation of donor-derived DCs to prevent donor-derived acute graft rejection and to promote tolerance induction. Other experimental evidence also supports a scientific basis for tolerance induction by DCs. Treatment of mice with fms-like tyrosine kinase

3 ligand (Flt-3L) causes increased numbers of DCs in the liver. It was predicted that a Flt3L-treated liver allograft would be quickly rejected, although livers are normally accepted without immunosuppressive therapy. Similarly, it was predicted that acute rejection of the liver allograft would occur if the recipients were treated with interleukin (IL)-12 or IL-2. What in fact happened when donor mice were treated with Flt-3L or when recipient mice were treated with IL-12 or IL-2? Both treatments dramatically reduced T-cell apoptosis. Thus, if T cells could be deleted by DCs, immunogenic tolerance could be achieved in transplant situations. Deletion of T cells could be achieved by:

1. Antigen-presenting cell-induced activation, causing cell death.
2. A blockade of costimulatory molecules on allogenic DCs, promoting the death and deletion of alloreactive T cells.
3. Introducing immature donor DCs, which when combined with anti-CD40 cause increased apoptotic death of graft-infiltrating cells.

Tolerance induction might be achieved by inducing both regulatory and anergic T cells. Immature donor DCs might deliver signal 1 in the absence of signal 2, which would eventually lead the production of regulatory T cells. These regulatory T cells produce IL-10 and transforming growth factor (TGF)-β, but low levels of IL-2, and no IL-4. The induction of regulatory T cells in this way has been shown in both mouse and human. Intravenous injection of humans with monocyte-derived immature DCs pulsed with influenza matrix protein should lead to the production of matrix-specific IL-10. In addition, constant stimulation of human cord blood T cells with immature DCs should lead to the production of IL-10-producing regulatory T cells. This has also been seen in a transplantation setting. Murine B-cell lineage-associated DCs derived from liver-resident progenitors have been shown to induce regulatory T cells in vitro, leading to the prolongation of allograft survival in vivo.

Immune tolerance could also be induced by immune deviation. The major damage in transplantation settings is probably done by T cells of Th1 phenotype. DCs are able to induce both Th1 and Th2 types of immune responses. If the immune response during transplantation can be skewed to the Th2 phenotype, that might lead to better survival of transplanted organs.

Although deletion of T cells, induction of regulatory T cells, and deviation of the immune response to the Th2 phenotype might result in immune tolerance, the timing of DC administration and the allograft operation would be critical for successful allograft acceptance. Bone marrow-derived DCs cultured with suboptimal doses of granulocyte-macrophage colony-stimulating factor (GM-CSF) retained an immature phenotype. When these DCs were administered to mice 7 days before transplantation, the allograft survived indefinitely. However, when DCs were administered 3, 14, or 28 days before transplantation, the allograft did not survive.

Blocking the maturation of DCs might also facilitate tolerance induction. DC maturation is mediated by nuclear translocation of nuclear factor (NF)-κB. Various drugs such as salicylates and corticosteroids block the maturation of DCs through this pathway. Immature DCs can also be produced by targeting the NF-κB pathway with antisense oligodeoxynucleotides (ODNs). Short ODNs with consensus binding sequences to NF-κb inhibit DC allostimulatory capacity by blocking NF-$\kappa\beta$ translocation. DCs treated with NF-$\kappa\beta$ ODNs for up to 36h and administered to fully allogenic recipients as a single intravenous dose 7 days before transplantation should prolong allograft survival.

DCs have also been manipulated by other agents to express IL-10, including cytotoxic T-lymphocyte-associated antigen (CTLA) 4, FasL, and TGF-β, as a method of producing tolerogenic DCs.

Chimerism and DCs

There is evidence that donor-derived passenger leukocytes, mainly DCs, can remain in the recipient for a long time, a state known as chimerism. Chimerism is the coexistence of cells from genetically different individuals. It is thought that chimerism of DCs from the donor (passenger leukocytes) and the recipient is very important. There are three types of chimerism: full chimerism, mixed chimerism, and microchimerism. In full chimerism, the entire recipient hematolymphoid system is replaced by that of the donor. In mixed chimerism, a functionally integrated immune system is composed of various proportions of hematolymphoid cells from the donor and recipient. Microchimerism is similar to mixed chimerism. It refers to trace populations of multilineage donor hematopoietic cells that persist in a few stable, unconditioned, long-term vascularized allograft recipients treated only with conventional immunosuppressive regimens. The presence of chimerism is thought to be associated with graft acceptance, and might even play a role in maintaining unresponsiveness to the graft. Since the advent of transplantation immunobiology, tolerance achieved by hematopoietic chimerism has been widely recognized as the ideal and most robust form of tolerance. A certain degree of chimerism is best achieved if the inoculum contains cells capable of self-renewal, for example, bone marrow cells. However, it is not possible to explain all of the tolerance of transplantation by chimerism. Individual patients were found that had apparently accepted an organ allograft, but who were not microchimeric, and, conversely, other patients were microchimeric, but rejected their allografts when immunosuppressive coverage was inadequate.

The robust tolerance associated with mixed chimerism is strictly dependent on the persistence of donor cells. In particular, successful mixed chimerism shows clonal deletion of self-reactive T cells in the thymus, which is mediated primarily by DCs. Donor DCs are able to migrate into the recipient thymic medulla and mediate negative selection of T cells potentially reactive against the allograft. Donor precursor cells can also mature into lymphoid or myeloid DCs and migrate into peripheral lymph nodes and into the interstitia of organs, where they can mediate immunogenic or tolerogenic reactions. The mixed chimerism approach to tolerance induction, which has been so successful in small experimental animals, has not gained widespread clinical acceptance.

The therapeutic efficacy of tolerance induction by DCs can be best explained in clinical situations of liver transplantation. Liver transplantation is unique in that HLA matching is not necessary even though it is absolutely necessary during the transplantation of most other organs. Spontaneous tolerance is induced after liver transplantation in many cases without immunosuppressive drugs. Moreover, liver transplantation can protect other organ grafts from the same donor transplanted in conjunction with the liver. This acceptance might be lost by removal of donor leukocytes prior to liver transplant. Part of the immunologically strange phenomena in liver transplantation might be explained by the characteristics of liver DCs. Liver DCs are inherently immature, and a considerable proportion of them express CD8α and secrete IL-10. These DCs have the features of tolerogenic DCs. Thus, transplantation of liver may induce tolerance because of the high proportion of immature and tolerogenic DCs in the liver. The liver is a hematopoietic organ, and may have the advantage of being a continuous source of donor hematopoietic cells. Donor-derived immature DCs may promote donor-specific tolerance induction. Large numbers of donor leukocytes present in a liver allograft cause overstimulation or abnormal early activation of recipient T cells, which leads to their exhaustive proliferation and deletional tolerance. Alloreactive host T-cell apoptosis in experimental liver transplantation is associated with tolerance, whereas less apoptosis is seen with rejection. Conceivably, the donor DC may play a role in inducing apoptosis in host T cells via death ligand–receptor pathways. Neutralization of IL-12 produced by liver-resident DCs restores long-term allograft survival and enhances alloreactive T-cell apoptosis. This suggests that suppression/inhibition of donor DC function promotes tolerance induction. The immature state of normal liver-derived DCs may be important in inherent liver tolerogenicity. Administration of liver DC progenitors prior to transplantation has been shown to increase allograft survival, although not to induce tolerance.

DC Subsets and Their Use in the Induction of Tolerance

Although DCs can be manipulated in animal models of transplantation, such manipulation is not simple or viable in human transplantation. However, different subsets of DCs with diverse functions are now beginning to be identified. For example, plasmacytoid DCs can be isolated from human peripheral blood. These cells are not good stimulators in allogenic MLRs, and they induce the Th2 phenotype after CD40 ligation. Granulocyte colony-stimulating factor-mobilized plasmacytoid DCs can induce tolerance. These DCs have been shown to participate in the prevention of host-versus-host diseases.

Control of Liver Allograft Rejection from Viral Infection

Liver transplantation is indicated in patients with liver failure due to fulminant hepatitis, liver cirrhosis, and hepatocellular carcinoma, the major causative agents of these diseases are hepatitis B virus (HBV) and hepatitis C virus (HCV). Although acute and chronic rejection of allografts constitute major problems in the context of transplantation, liver allografts might be rejected due to a flare-up of hepatitis virus infections in patients chronically infected with these viruses. Although HBV and HCV are presumed to be hepatotrophic, these viruses can be detected in many extrahepatic sites, including bone marrow and peripheral blood mononuclear cells. When liver is transplanted to patients with chronic HBV infection, they are given high titers of costly hyperimmune γ-globulins for the rest of their lives. In addition, some of these patients also receive immunosuppressive therapy. Recently, it was shown that injection of HBsAg-pulsed DCs induced anti-HBs, the protective antibody of HBV infection, in immunosuppressed HBV transgenic mice, a murine model of HBV carrier status. Immunosuppression was achieved in HBV transgenic mice by daily injection of tacrolimus. Although this procedure would solve the problem of flare-ups of HBV after transplantation into chronic HBV carriers, the challenging question is whether it would reduce the rejection of liver allografts by patients.

Concluding Remarks

It is evident that DCs play a dominant role in the rejection of allografts. Accumulated evidence also suggests that DCs are involved in the process of peripheral T-cell tolerance, which may increase the likelihood of allograft acceptance. Techniques have also been developed to isolate or enrich abundant amounts of DCs in vitro, and the various DC subsets can also be produced in vitro. Advances in vectorology and gene therapy will allow the production of tolerogenic DCs. All this experimental evidence strongly suggests that it might be feasible to use DC-based alloantigen-specific T-cell hyporesponsiveness to improve allograft acceptance. However, one of the main obstacles is that we have very little information regarding the mechanism of induction of peripheral T-cell tolerance in the normal steady state. Moreover, very little is known about the cellular and molecular events underlying the maintenance of this tolerance. A thorough understanding of the induction and maintenance of tolerance to self- and nonself-antigens in steady state is needed.

Recommended Readings

Coates PT, Thomson AW (2002) Dendritic cells, tolerance induction and transplant outcome. Am J Transplant 2:299–307

Demetris AJ, Murase N, Starzl TE (1992) Donor dendritic cells after liver and heart allotransplantation under short-term immunosuppression. Lancet 339:1610

Dhodapkar MV, Steinman RM, Krasovsky J (2001) Antigen-specific inhibition of effector T cell function in humans after injection of immature dendritic cells. J Exp Med 193: 233–238

Hackstein H, Morelli AE, Thomson AW (2001) Designer dendritic cells for tolerance induction: guided not misguided missiles. Trends Immunol 22:437–442

Lau AH, Thomson AW (2003) Dendritic cells and immune regulation in the liver. Gut 52: 307–314

Lechler R, Ng WF, Steinman RM (2001) Dendritic cells in transplantation–friend or foe? Immunity 14:357–368

Morellia AE, Hackstein H, Thomson AW (2001) Potential of tolerogenic dendritic cells for transplantation. Semin Immunol 13:323–335

8. Follicular Dendritic Cells

General Considerations

Outline and Definition

Follicular dendritic cells (FDCs) take their name from the presence of dendritic processes on these cells. However, FDCs are a completely different type of cell from the dendritic cells (DCs) that are the subject of most of the chapters in this book. The ontogeny of FDCs is different from that of antigen-presenting DCs. DCs are known to originate in the bone marrow, and progenitors and precursors of DCs are known, but the origin of FDCs is unknown. DCs are widely distributed throughout the entire body, but FDCs exhibit a highly specialized type of distribution. They are localized in the light zones of the germinal centers in the secondary lymphoid follicles. The functions of FDCs have to do with B cells; especially, they stimulate the memory B cells. However, the main function of antigen-presenting DCs is to present antigens to T cells, although DCs are capable of performing a variety of functions as part of both the innate and adaptive immune responses.

FDCs have some characteristic features: They are resistant to irradiation and have a long half-life. In addition, FDCs have three features that are useful for distinguishing these cells from other immune cells: (1) FDCs exhibit a dendritic morphology; (2) the distribution of FDCs is restricted to the light zones of germinal centers in the lymphoid follicles; and (3) they trap and retain immune complexes on their surfaces for long periods. Surface antigens such as CD21, CD35, CD23, R4/23, and KiM4 can be detected on FDCs, but they are not FDC-specific.

Origin of FDCs

The exact nature of the cells that give rise to FDCs remains an enigma. Many cytokines and receptors join in the formation of lymphoid follicles, which are FDC networks. Mice deficient in tumor necrosis factor (TNF)-α, lymphotoxin (LT)-α or LT-β lack or have severely underdeveloped FDC networks. In addition, mice lacking expression of the tumor necrosis factor receptor (TNFR) I or the LT-β receptor are also unable to produce FDC networks. Interleukin (IL)-6 is another cytokine produced by FDCs that is important for proper expansion of the germinal center reaction. IL-6 produced by FDCs regulates molecules produced by other cell types in order to maintain the stepwise progression of high-affinity humoral responses. Soluble IL-13 receptor from germinal center B cells signal the FDCs to produce IL-6. FDCs also express molecules, other than immune complex receptors, which are pivotal in driving the high-affinity antibody response.

Functions of FDCs

FDCs are identified by immunostaining with specific antibodies. It is also possible to isolate and culture FDCs for functional characterization. FDCs are central players in humoral immunity. They are found in the B-cell regions of all secondary lymphoid tissue, and they have the unique capacity to trap and retain immune complexes for long periods. FDCs act as nurse cells for B cells, so they are potent B-cell accessory cells. Germinal centers are characterized by rapidly proliferating, somatically mutating B cells, and FDCs play an important role in regulating events in this special microenvironment. Most B cells in the germinal centers appear to die and be taken up by tingle body macrophages. However, some germinal center B cells compete for and bind the antigens on the FDCs and emerge as antibody-forming cells that produce high-affinity antibodies. Some of these cells might be converted to memory B cells with high-affinity receptors. Antigens retained on FDC networks in the form of immune complexes have long been known to provide signals to germinal center B cells. Germinal center B cells associate with and internalize antigens trapped on immune complex-coated bodies (iccosomes). The function of FDCs is to establish a suitable microenvironment to support the expansion and affinity maturation of centroblasts, where immune complexes displayed on the surface of FDCs engage the B-cell receptors of antigen-stimulated B cells.

In the germinal centers of the lymphoid follicles, $CD4^+$, $CD11c^+$, $CD3^-$ dendritic cells, so-called germinal center dendritic cells (GCDCs) are present. FDCs are also found in the same region (Fig. 8.1). GCDCs are present in both the dark and light zones of germinal centers in human tonsils, spleen, and lymph nodes. They may induce or sustain the response of memory T cells in germinal centers, and maintain the germinal center reaction during secondary T-cell-dependent responses of B cells. However, the relationship between FDCs and GCDCs is not clear.

T cells, B cells, plasmacytoid DCs, and other cells come through high endothelial venules into the T-cell area (Fig. 8.1). In the germinal centers, antigen-specific T cells are activated by interdigitating dendritic cells in the T-cell area. These T cells migrate to the follicle border, where they activate antigen-specific B cells. Some B cells become antibody-producing plasma cells, whereas other B cells migrate to the primary follicles, where they initiate formation of the germinal center. Antigens and FDCs select B cells bearing high-affinity B cell receptors. Low-affinity B cells undergo apoptosis. Antigen-dependent T cell-mediated reactions induce isotype switching and the formation of plasma cells and memory cells.

FDCs in Pathological Conditions

Viral Hepatitis

There are several reports of the formation of lymphoid follicles in the portal spaces in patients with various chronic liver diseases, including autoimmune hepatitis,

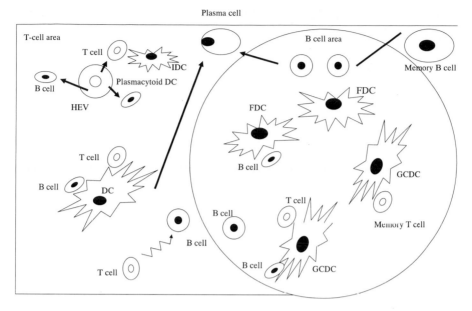

Fig. 8.1. Follicular dendritic cells (FDCs) are detected in the B-cell area of the lymphoid follicles. Memory B cells and plasma cells are seen in close proximity to plasma cells. Germinal center dendritic cells (GCDCs) lie close to FDCs and may interact with B cells and T cells. *IDC*, interdigitating dendritic cell; *HEV*, high endothelial venule; *IDC*, interdigitating cells

primary biliary cirrhosis, and viral hepatitis. The presence of lymphoid follicles in patients with liver diseases influenced some hepatologists to call these diseases "follicular hepatitis," a condition in which chronic viral hepatitis is associated with the formation of lymphoid follicles. In chronic viral hepatitis, portal tracts are infiltrated by mononuclear cells. Although the bulk of these cells are lymphocytes, other immunocytes have also been detected in these follicles. Lymphoid follicles are seen in about 10% of patients with chronic hepatitis B. In one study, hepatitis B virus surface antigen (HBsAg) was detected by immunohistochemistry in the hepatocytes as well as in the center of the follicles in about half of the patients (Fig. 8.2). By immune electron microscopy, signals for HBsAg and pre-S2 antigens of hepatitis B virus (HBV) have been detected in the dendritic processes of FDCs (Fig. 8.3). It is possible that HBsAg or pre-S2 antigens are retained on the surfaces of FDCs for prolonged periods. HBsAg has also been detected in the lymphoid follicles of the spleen.

The incidence of lymphoid follicles has been proved to be significantly higher in patients with chronic hepatitis due to hepatitis C virus (HCV) than in those with HBV. However, no one has studied FDCs and the presence of HCV-associated proteins in patients with chronic HCV infection.

Human Immunodeficiency Virus

An association between retroviruses and FDCs seems to have profound consequences for both host and pathogen. Soon after a patient becomes infected with human

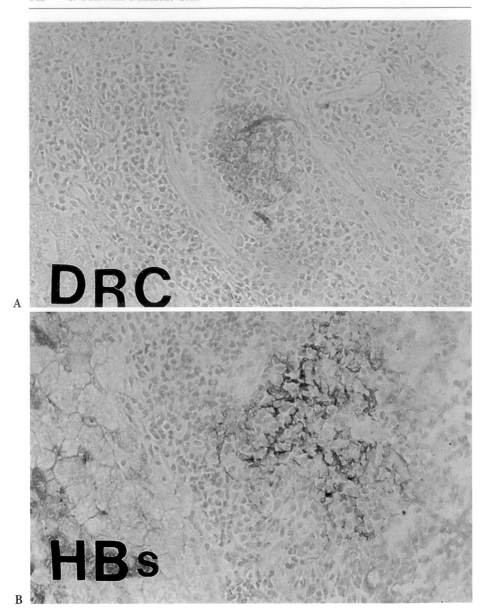

Fig. 8.2. A Localization of FDCs in the lymphoid follicles in liver tissue from patients with chronic hepatitis B. **B** Hepatitis B surface antigen (HBsAg) was localized in the same area of the liver tissue that contained FDCs in the consecutive section of the liver biopsy specimen. *DRC*, dendritic reticullar cell. Original magnification ×300. Brownish color indicate staining for dendritic reticular cells and HBsAg

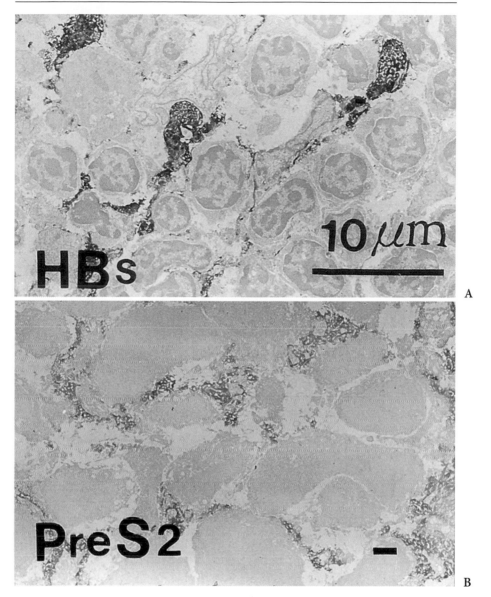

Fig. 8.3A,B. An immune electron microscope view showing the expression of HBsAg (**A**) and pre-S2 antigen (**B**) on the dendritic processes of FDCs. Black signals indicate HBs and pre S2

immunodeficiency virus (HIV) 1, these viruses are trapped on FDCs, perhaps causing a potent reservoir of infectious virus adjacent to highly susceptible CD4-bearing T cells to become established. FDCs trap and retain HIV antigens in their native state for many months. HIV particles trapped on FDCs can be observed until the follicular network is destroyed. In the progressive stages of HIV infection, HIV-loaded FDCs migrate into the lymphatic circulation. Active HIV infection is largely confined to sites surrounding FDCs, suggesting that this microenvironment is highly conducive to the persistence of infection. FDCs maintain HIV infectivity and trapped viruses can cause infection even in the presence of neutralizing antibodies. FDCs also contribute signals to the germinal center microenvironment, which may induce an increased rate of replication of HIV. Because of virus trapping, previously trapped antigens on FDCs are lost and cannot be retrapped; shortly afterward, specific antibody responses to these antigens become markedly impaired. Eventually, the FDC network is destroyed during HIV infection, although the underlying cause is unknown. FDCs appear to play a role in pathogenesis after initial HIV infection and seeding of the secondary lymphoid tissue have occurred. There are no reports of interaction between FDCs and DCs or, especially, GCDCs in the lymphoid follicles under physiological or pathological conditions.

FDCs and Prions

Prion diseases are characterized by the accumulation of infectious particles known as protease-resistant prions (PrPres). Abundant PrPres are detected, before the appearance of the clinical signs of the disease, in the germinal centers of tonsils and appendixes of patients affected with Creutzfeldt–Jakob disease. FDCs could be the site of PrPres retention and amplification, or perhaps FDCs produce PrPres. FDCs represent a potential target for prophylactic or therapeutic intervention in transmissible spongiform encephalopathies.

FDCs and Autoimmunity

Autoimmune diseases, especially organ-specific autoimmune diseases such as rheumatoid arthritis, Hashimoto's disease, and primary biliary cirrhosis, show the formation of secondary lymphoid follicles in the affected organs. FDCs have been localized in these follicles. FDCs in the germinal center of the thyroid lesion of Hashimoto's disease have thyroglobulin and antibody complexes. In primary biliary cirrhosis, FDCs in the regional lymph node of liver express pyruvate dehydrogenase complex. Probably, FDCs play a role in the production of autoantibodies. However, the actual functions of FDCs in autoimmune diseases are still unknown.

FDCs and Tumors

FDCs in the neoplastic nodules of follicular lymphomas retain their immune complex-trapping mechanism and their expression of complement receptors. However, most diffuse lymphomas have irregular, distorted, and disappearing FDC networks. Castleman's disease shows abnormal FDC networks. There are few reports on the characterization and functioning of FDCs in malignant lesions.

Tumors showing differentiation toward FDCs have been documented, but tumors of FDCs are very uncommon. Most of these tumors are found in the lymph nodes, or rarely in extranodal sites, including stomach, colon, liver, thyroid, breast, and the oral cavity. The diagnosis of FDC tumors should be based on the recognition of FDCs, which exhibit distinctive histological features. However, a definite diagnosis requires confirmation with immunohistochemical studies. FDC tumors show immune reactivity with some of the markers for FDCs, for example, CD21, CD35, R4/23, Ki-M4, and FDC-M4p. Approximately 12% of all reported cases of FDC tumors are associated with Epstein-Barr virus, because CD21 is the receptor for this virus. However, the role of this virus in the pathogenesis of FDC tumors remains to be established.

Concluding Remarks

FDCs play a central role in humoral immunity. Lymphoid follicles with germinal centers are formed in many organs in patients suffering from chronic infections. FDCs form an extensive network in these germinal centers. Understanding the role of FDCs in the regulation of B-cell function and humoral immunity would provide insight into disease pathogeneses.

It is ironic that even though antigen-presenting DCs also regulate the function of B lymphocytes and are present in lymphoid follicles, a working relationship between these two cell types has not been shown.

Recommended Readings

Burton GF, Keele BF, Estes, et al. (2002) Follicular dendritic cell contributions to HIV pathogenesis. Semin Immunol 14:275–284

Grouard G, Durand I, Filgueira L, et al. (1996) Dendritic cells capable of stimulating T cells in germinal centres. Nature 384:364–367

Tew JG, Wu J, Fakher M, et al. (2001) Follicular dendritic cells: beyond the necessity of T-cell help. Trends Immunol 22:361–367

Glossary

- **Anergy**
  Failure to make an immune response following stimulation with potential antigens.
- **Antigen presentation**
  The process by which certain cells in the body (antigen-presenting cells) express antigens on their cell surface in a form recognizable by lymphocytes.
- **APCs (Antigen-presenting cells)**
  A variety of cell types that carry antigens in a form for presentation to lymphocytes. Only DCs can present antigens to naive lymphocytes.
- **Antigen processing**
  The conversion of an antigen within antigen-presenting cells to a form that can be recognized by lymphocytes.
- **Antigen recognition**
  An inherent capacity of antigen-presenting cells that enables them to sense the presence of antigens or microbial agents.
- **Apoptosis**
  Programmed cell death, which involves nuclear fragmentation and condensation of cytoplasm, plasma membranes, and organelles into apoptotic bodies.
- **B 220**
  Common leukocyte antigen that is expressed on different types of cells including some DCs.
- **BAFF (B-cell activating factor belonging to the TNF family)**
  A critical survival/maturation factor for peripheral B cells. DC derived BAFF is a key molecule by which DCs directly regulate human B-cell proliferative responses to T-cell-independent stimuli.
- **BDCA (Blood dendritic cell antigen)**
  Antigen expressed on circulating peripheral blood DCs. Four BDCA antigens (BDCA 1–4) have been reported.
- **Birbeck granule**
  Rod-shaped or tennis-racket-shaped trilaminar cytoplasmic structure in Langerhans cells. Birbeck granules are present in immature and semi-matured Langerhans cells, but are reduced and lost upon their maturation.
- **CCR (CC chemokine receptor)**
  Receptor for CC chemokines. The expression of various CCRs on different immunocytes, including DCs, determines their migration to tissues expressing the ligands of their receptors.

- **CD1a**
Member of the immunoglobulin supergene family. Expressed on a subset of blood DCs and Langerhans cells.
- **CD11b**
Also known as Mac-1. A subset of DCs express this myeloid marker.
- **CD11c**
Also known as leukocyte surface antigen p150/90. A member of the integrin family, it is expressed on most DC populations in mouse and human.
- **CD16 (FcγRIII), CD32 (FcγRII), CD64 (FcγRI)**
These are Fc gamma receptors. DCs use these receptors for phagocytosis.
- **CD18**
A member of the β-2 integrin family, regarded as the beta subunit of CD11a, CD11b, and CD11c. CD18 acts in conjunction with members of the CD11 family.
- **CD21**
This is a receptor for Epstein-Barr virus.
- **CD23**
Low-affinity IgE receptor. Regulates IgE synthesis. Triggers the release of various cytokines and immune mediators from human monocytes (TNF-α, IL-1, IL-6, and GM-CSF).
- **CD34**
Expressed on hematopoietic progenitor cells. Its cellular function includes cell–cell adhesion. As the differentiation of hematopoietic progenitor cells progresses, CD34 is gradually lost. DCs can be obtained directly from cultures of CD34$^+$ hematopoietic progenitor cells.
- **CD35**
Also called immune adherence receptor. On leukocytes and tissue sources, CD35 mediates adherence of C4b/C3b coated particles in preparation for phagocytosis. Phagocytosis most often requires the cooperation of CD35 with complement receptor type 3 (CR3, CD11b/CD18) and the Fcγ complement receptor type-1.
- **CD36**
Scavenger receptor for oxidized products. It is also capable of recognition and phagocytosis of apoptotic cells.
- **CD40**
Expressed on DCs, and its ligation with CD40L on T cells induces the activation and maturation of DCs.
- **CD45RA**
Common leukocyte antigen, CD45, is a tyrosine phosphatase. It has several isoforms, and the CD45RA isoform is expressed on naive T cells.
- **CD46**
Cofactor for factor I proteolytic cleavage of C3b and C4b. It acts as a receptor for measles virus.
- **CD51**
Vitronectin receptor. It encodes integrin alpha chain V. αvβ3 is the most studied integrin of this family. This receptor functions during internalization of apoptotic bodies.

- **CD62L**
This ligand mediates homing of immunocytes to high endothelial venules of the peripheral lymphoid tissue and leukocyte rolling on activated endothelium at inflammatory sites. It is expressed on plasmacytoid DCs.
- **CD68**
Expressed on a population of DCs (plasmacytoid DCs) and macrophages.
- **CD80 and CD86**
Costimulatory molecules those are present on antigen-presenting cells. These molecules provide costimulation for T-cell activation via ligation with CD28 and suppression via ligation with CTLA-4.
- **CD83**
A member of the immunoglobulin superfamily. Expressed on mature DCs from different sources.
- **CD95 (Fas)**
A molecule expressed on a variety of cells that acts as a target for ligation by FasL. This molecule is involved in apoptosis.
- **CD123**
Interleukin-3 receptor. The expression of CD123 on plasmacytoid DCs but not on myeloid DCs has made it possible to isolate plasmacytoid DCs from peripheral blood.
- **Central tolerance**
Tolerance of T cells or B cells induced during their development in the thymus or bone marrow.
- **Chimerism**
The coexistence of cells from genetically different subjects.
- **c-kit (CD117)**
Member of the immunoglobulin supergene family. A receptor for stem cell factor, required for the early development of leukocytes.
- **CLA (Cutaneous leukocyte antigen)**
Expressed on Langerhans cells that colonize the skin. It is a coreceptor for E-selectin (CD62 E), which is expressed on the surface of activated endothelial cells. Expression of CLA allows the attachment and transendothelial migration of circulating cells to the dermis.
- **CLP (Common myeloid progenitors)**
Progenitors that give rise to cells of myeloid lineages.
- **CMP (Common lymphoid progenitors)**
Progenitors that give rise to cells of lymphoid lineages.
- **CMRF**
Markers on human DCs expressed during their differentiation and maturation.
- **Costimuli**
Signals required for the activation of lymphocytes in addition to the antigen-specific signal delivered via their antigen receptors. CD28 is an important costimulatory molecule for T cells and CD40 for B cells.
- **Conditioned DCs**
DCs activated by T helper cells (DC conditioning). These conditioned DCs can stimulate cytotoxic T cells without the presence of T helper cells.

- **Cryptopatch**
  Cryptopatches are solitary lymphoid structures found in murine and human gut. These were first identified in gut-associated murine lymphoid tissues, where the generation of IL-7-dependent lympho-hematopoietic progenitors for T- and/or B-cell descendants may begin. Cryptopatches also contain DCs.
- **CTLA (Cytotoxic T-lymphocyte-associated antigen)**
  An adhesion molecule in T cells, binds to CD80 and CD86 on DCs.
- **Danger signal**
  A signal that induces an immune response. Danger signals can be provided by cytokines, inflammatory mucosal milieu, microbial agents, and other nonself entities.
- **33D1**
  A rat monoclonal antibody that detects DCs in the murine spleen.
- **DC progenitors**
  Hematopoietic progenitor cells capable of producing DCs or DC precursors. These cells retain the capacity for proliferation.
- **DC precursors**
  These cells are more committed to become DCs than DC progenitors. Some DC precursors are well differentiated; however, others have not been well characterized. Monocytes are the most common DC precursors.
- **DC-SIGN (Dendritic cell-specific ICAM-grabbing nonintegrin, CD207)**
  DC-SIGN is a mannose-specific C-type lectin expressed by DCs. DC-SIGN binds to ICAM-3 on T lymphocytes, and plays an important role in the activation of T lymphocytes. DC-SIGN acts as a coreceptor for HIV, and the virus may remain bound to DC-SIGN for protracted periods.
- **DEC-205**
  205 kDa mouse glycoprotein lectin that is recognized by the monoclonal antibody NLDC-145. This molecule is important for the trapping of antigens by DCs. Abundant expression of DEC-205 is seen in mouse Langerhans cells and interdigitating dendritic cells. Very low levels of DEC-205 are expressed by B cells, activated macrophages, and epithelial cells of the intestine and bronchia.
- **DC1, DC2**
  Subsets of human DCs based on the expression of CD11c and CD123 on their precursor populations. Generally, DC1 and DC2 induce Th1 and Th2 polarization, respectively, but their polarization capacities depend on the nature and type of the stimulus.
- **Exhausted DCs**
  DCs stimulated for a prolonged time that become nonresponsive to a stimulus are regarded as exhausted DCs. However, the exhausted DCs might become functional again if they are cultured in media free of the original stimulus.
- **Extrathymic differentiation of T cells**
  Differentiation of T cells outside the thymus.
- **Fc receptor**
  A type of phagocytic receptor. Antigens, microbes, and apoptotic cells may be internalized by cells having these receptors. There are different types of Fc receptors.
- **FDC (Follicular dendritic cell)**
  A novel cell type with dendritic morphology. These cells are localized in the light zone of germinal centers. FDCs possibly trap and retain antigen/antibody complexes.

- **Flt-3L (fms-like tyrosine kinase receptor 3 ligand)**
  Flt-3L stimulates the proliferation of stem and progenitor cells and including DCs by binding to the Flt-3 receptor, which is a type III receptor tyrosine kinase member of the PDGF family. Flt-3L induces proliferation of both myeloid and lymphoid DCs.
- **$\gamma\delta$ T cells**
  A minor subset of T cells that expresses the $\gamma\delta$ form of the T-cell receptor. Most $\gamma\delta$ T cells are differentiated in extrathymic organs. For example, one third of liver sinusoidal T cells are $\gamma\delta$ T cells.
- **Gr-1**
  A granulocyte marker also found on plasmacytoid DCs.
- **Germinal centers**
  Areas of secondary lymphoid tissue in which B-cell differentiation and antibody class switching occurs.
- **GCDC (Germinal center dendritic cells (GCDC)**
  DCs presenting in both dark and light zones of germinal centers in human tonsils, spleen, and lymph nodes, and also associated with germinal center T cells. GCDCs are $CD4^+$, $CD11c^-$, and $CD3^-$.
- **GM-CSF (Granulocyte-macrophage colony-stimulating factor)**
  Required for differentiation of DCs from DC progenitors, DC precursors, and cells of myeloid lineages.
- **gp (Glycoprotein)**
  Expressed on different strains of human immune deficiency virus.
- **HBV (Hepatitis B virus), HCV (Hepatitis C virus)**
  HBV is a DNA virus of the hepadna virus family. HCV is a member of flavivirus family. Both HBV and HCV cause acute as well as chronic liver diseases including liver cirrhosis and hepatocellular carcinoma.
- **HEV (High endothelial venule)**
  An area of venules from which lymphocytes and other cells migrate into the lymph nodes.
- **ICAM-1 (CD54), ICAM-2 (CD102) and ICAM-3 (CD50) (Intercellular adhesion molecules)**
  Cell-surface molecules found on a variety of leucocytes and nonhematogenous cells.
- **Iccosomes**
  Immune complexes in the form of small inclusion bodies found in follicular dendritic cells.
- **ILT (Immunoglobulin-like transcript)**
  Marker for DC precursor cells. Lin^-, $ILT3^+$, and $ILT1^+$ cells appear to correspond to the $CD11c^+$ myeloid DC precursors, whereas Lin^-, $ILT3^+$, $ILT1^-$ cells appear to be essentially equivalent to the $CD11c^-$ plasmacytoid DCs. A hallmark of the $ILT3^+$, $ILT1^-$, and $CD11c^-$ subsets is their striking production of type-I interferon following viral infection.
- **Immature DCs**
  DCs expressing low levels of costimulatory molecules and with a potent antigen-capturing capacity.

- **Innate immunity**
  Immune response that is induced immediately after the entry of microbial agents. Innate immunity is very quick, and various leukocytes act as effector cells of innate immunity.
- **Interleukin (IL)**
  A group of mediators that regulate the growth and proliferation of different cells both positively and negatively. There are several interleukins.
- **IL-3**
  This cytokine induces the maturation of human peripheral blood plasmacytoid DCs in vitro.
- **IL-4**
  This cytokine is used to generate DCs from human monocytes.
- **IL-6**
  A pleiotropic cytokine, whose functions include costimulation of B cells, development of CTLs, and enhancement of survival of naive T cells. It can also suppress several immunological functions.
- **IL-10**
  An immunoregulatory cytokine. It acts directly on mouse Th cells. In humans, it acts via APCs. It facilitates the generation and survival of CTLs. Usually attributed to Th2 polarization. Tolerogenic DCs can be produced by culturing DCs with IL-10.
- **IL-12**
  Most DCs can produce IL-12 after various stimuli. It is a key cytokine for the development and maintenance of cellular immunity. It induces Th1 polarization. Important survival factor for CTL, Th1, and DCs.
- **IL-13**
  Can be used to generate DCs in spite of the presence of IL-4. Causes maturation of monocyte-derived DCs grown in GM-CSF and IL-4.
- **IL-15**
  Produced by LCs, DDCs, and mature monocyte- and $CD34^+$-derived DCs. IL-15 induces the proliferation of T cells and promotes the generation of CTLs.
- **IL-18**
  Also called IFN-γ-inducing factor. Acts synergistically with IL-12. Enhances production of IL-1, IFN-γ, GM-CSF, and IL-13. Increases in mature DCs.
- **IDC (Interdigitating dendritic cells)**
  DCs in the T-cell areas of peripheral lymphoid organs such as the spleen, lymph node, and Peyer's patch. These cells express MHC II, invariant chain, high levels of self-antigens, accessory molecules such as CD40 and CD86, a multilectin receptor for antigen presentation called DEC-205, the integrin CD11c, several antigens within the endocytic system and, in the human system, the molecules S100b, CD83, and p55.
- **IFN-α (Interferon-α)**
  Also called type-1 IFN. IFN-α has potent antiviral potential. Plasmacytoid DCs produce abundant amounts of IFN-α with viral stimulation.
- **IRF (Interferon regulatory factor)**
  Members of the IRF family induce the sequential expression of type-1 IFN genes. Viruses, DNA motifs, and double-stranded RNA might activate different IRF molecules. The expression of IRF molecules is regulated during maturation and activation of DCs.

- **Killer DCs**
  DCs expressing FasL. They are able to kill target cells.
- **KiM4 and R4/23**
  Antibodies that react with antigens on some follicular dendritic cells.
- **Langerhans' cells**
  Antigen-presenting cells of the skin expressing Birbeck granules and langerin.
- **Langerin**
  A type II Ca^{2+}-dependent lectin displaying mannose-binding specificity. Langerin colocalizes with Birbeck granules. Transfection of langerin cDNA into fibroblasts results in Birbeck granule formation.
- **Lineage**
  Markers that are present on myeloid or lymphoid cells. In general, DCs are lineage negative, but some DCs express variable amounts of lineage markers.
- **Lymphoid DCs**
  DCs expressing CD8 antigen in the mouse.
- **LT (Lymphotoxin)**
  Ligand of the TNF-α receptor family. LT has both α and β subunits. Mice deficient in either LT-α or LT-β lack or have a severely underdeveloped FDC network.
- **MIIC (MHC class II-rich compartment)**
  Specialized late endosomal MHC class II-rich compartment vesicles of antigen-presenting cells. DCs store the intact antigen in an MIIC until the receipt of an activation signal for the induction of the immune response. Constitutive peptide-MIIC class II complex generation occurs in immature DCs, which may induce peripheral tolerance
- **MIF (Macrophage migration inhibition factor)**
  A group of peptides produced by lymphocytes, macrophages, and DCs, capable of inhibiting random migration of macrophages.
- **MIP-3 (Macrophage inflammatory protein-3)**
  There are two MIP-3 proteins: MIP-3α and MIP-3β. The receptors for MIP-3α and MIP-3β are expressed on immature and mature DCs, respectively.
- **Myeloid DCs**
  Mouse DCs that are $CD8^-$ and $CD11b^+$. In human $CD11c^+$ DCs are regarded as myeloid DCs.
- **NIPC (Natural interferon-producing Cell)**
  Plasmacytoid DCs which are $CD11c^-$, $CD4^+$, $CD123^+$. They produce abundant amounts of type-1 interferon after viral stimulation.
- **Nef, gag, gp120**
  These are antigens related to HIV.
- **NK (Natural killer) cells**
  A group of cells with intrinsic ability to recognize and destroy some virally infected cells and tumor cells.
- **NKT cell**
  Lymphocyte having markers of both T and NK cells. These cells express Vα24 receptor. NKT cells can recognize α-galactosylceramide through binding with the CD1d molecule.

- **NF-κB (Nuclear factor κB)**
  A transcription factor that plays a central role in immunological processes by regulating genes involved in the immune and inflammatory responses.
- **NO (Nitric oxide)**
  Produced by a variety of cells including DCs. It regulates the immune response both positively and negatively.
- **ODN (Oligodeoxynucleotide)**
  Activates immune cells, including DCs, through the NF-κB signaling pathway. ODNs and decoy ODNs might regulate the immune response positively and negatively, respectively.
- **Oral tolerance**
  Induction of immune tolerance by ingestion of food antigens via the oral route.
- **PALS (Periarteriolar lymphoid sheath)**
  Present in the lymphoid tissues. A particular type of DC is localized in this lymphoid tissue compartment.
- **Peripheral tolerance**
  A state of specific immunological unresponsiveness.
- **Peyer's patches**
  Collections of lymphoid cells in the wall of the gut that form secondary lymphoid tissue.
- **Plasmacytoid dendritic cell**
  Large lymphocyte having a plasma cell-like appearance. These cells produce abundant amounts of type-I interferon after viral stimulation. They can also act as professional antigen-presenting cells.
- **Professional APC**
  Antigen-presenting cells able to stimulate and induce proliferation of naive T cells.
- **RelB**
  A subunit of the nuclear factor (NF)-κB transcription factor. It is expressed on different DC populations and implicated in DC differentiation and maturation.
- **SLC (Secondary lymphoid chemokine)**
  This is a chemotactic cytokine highly expressed within lymphoid organs. It binds to CCR7 and is a potent attractant of T cells and mature DCs.
- **SCF (Stem cell factor)**
  SCF is an essential hemopoietic progenitor cell growth factor with proliferative and anti-apoptotic functions.
- **S100 proteins**
  Intracytoplasmic calcium-binding proteins, expressed on some DCs as well as on other lymphoid cells, nerve cells, chondrocytes, lipid cells, and melanocytes.
- **TAA (Tumor-associated antigen)**
  Peptide antigen expressed by tumor cells but not by normal cells. TAA can induce TAA-specific immunity in some circumstances.
- **TAP (Transporter associated with antigen processing)**
  This pathway is required for the intracellular transport of antigens to MHC class I molecules.

- **TLR (Toll-like receptor)**
  The TLRs are type 1 transmembrane receptors that possess an extracellular leucine-rich repeat domain and a cytoplasmic domain homologous to that of the interleukin 1 receptor (IL-1R) family. Different TLRs are expressed by different DC populations.
- **Thy 1.1 and Thy 1.2**
  Markers of T lymphocytes in the mouse.
- **Thymic dendritic cell**
  DCs in thymus are BP-1$^+$, CD11c$^+$, DEC-205$^+$, M342$^+$ and CD8$^+$. Thymic DCs play a principal role in central tolerance.
- **TNF (Tumor necrosis factor)**
  A cytokine released by activated macrophages and other cells that is structurally related to lymphotoxin released by activated T cells.
- **TNFR (TNF receptor)**
  There are two TNFR, TNFRI (p55) and TNFRII (p75). Both of them can induce signal transduction.
- **TGF (Transforming growth factor)**
  TGFs comprise a group of cytokines identified by their ability to promote fibroblast growth. They are generally immunosuppressive. TGF-β promotes growth of LCs from monocytes.
- **Tolerogenic DCs**
  DCs manipulated in vitro exploit the same mechanisms that normal DCs employ to induce/maintain peripheral and central tolerance under steady-state conditions. Tolerogenic DCs may prove to be an invaluable tool for therapy in allograft rejection, autoimmune diseases, or allergies.
- **VCAM (Vascular cell adhesion molecule)**
  Expressed on endothelial cells and related to allergic manifestations.

Bibliography

Sources of figures are shown in boldface in parentheses.

1986–1996

Kanaoka M, Kumon I, Michitaka K, Onji M, Nadano S, Ohta Y (1986) An electron microscopic study of follicular hepatitis. J Clin Electron Microscopy 19:559–560

Yamashita Y (1986) Studies on the stimulatory function of peripheral blood monocytes against T cell blastogenesis and the activity of suppressor mechanism in patients with chronic liver diseases. Acta Hepatol Jpn 27:736–743

Yamashita Y (1986) Enumeration of I region associated (Ia) antigen bearing monocyte in chronic liver diseases. Acta Hepatol Jpn 27:924–933

Kumon I, Onji M, Nadano S, Kanaoka M, Ohta Y (1989) Detection of hepatitis B surface antigen in lymphoid follicle in patients with chronic hepatitis type B. Gastroenterol Jpn 24:738 (**Fig. 8.2, Fig. 8.3**)

Kumon I (1992) In situ characterization of mononuclear cell phenotype in intrahepatic lymphoid follicle in patients with chronic viral hepatitis. Gastroenterol Jpn 27:638–645 (**Fig. 8.2, Fig. 8.3**)

Akbar SMF, Onji M, Inaba K, Yamamura K-I, Ohta Y (1993) Low responsiveness of hepatitis B virus-transgenic mice in antibody response to T-cell dependent antigen: defect in antigen-presenting activity of dendritic cells. Immunology 78:468–475

Akbar SMF, Inaba K, Onji M (1996) Upregulation of MHC class II antigen on dendritic cells from hepatitis B virus transgenic mice by interferon-gamma: abrogation of immune response defect to a T-cell-dependent antigen. Immunology 87:519–527

1997

Akbar SMF, Kajino K, Tanimoto K, Kurose K, Masumoto T, Michitaka K, Horiike N, Onji M (1997) Placebo-controlled trial of vaccination with hepatitis B virus surface antigen in hepatitis B virus transgenic mice. J Hepatol 26:131–137

Kurose K, Akbar SMF, Yamamoto K, Onji M (1997) Production of antibody to hepatitis B surface antigen (anti-HBs) by murine hepatitis B virus carriers: neonatal tolerance versus antigen presentation by dendritic cells. Immunology 92:494–500

1998

Akbar SMF, Onji M (1998) Hepatitis B virus (HBV) transgenic mice as an investigative tool to study immunopathology during HBV infection. Int J Exp Pathol 79:279–291

Hiasa Y, Horiike N, Akbar SMF, Saito I, Miyamura T, Matsuura Y, Onji M (1998) Low stimulatory capacity of lymphoid dendritic cells expressing hepatitis C virus genes. Biochem Biophys Res Commun 249:90–95

Shinomiya M, Masumoto T, Nadano S, Akbar SMF, Onji M (1998) Lymphoid dendritic cells in the liver of patients with primary biliary cirrhosis and its mouse model. Hepatol Res 1:84–94 **(Fig. 5.2)**

Yamamoto K, Akbar SMF, Masumoto T, Onji M (1998) Increased nitric oxide (NO) production by antigen-presenting dendritic cells is responsible for low allogeneic mixed leucocyte reaction (MLR) in primary biliary cirrhosis (PBC). Clin Exp Immunol 114: 94–101 **(Fig. 5.4)**

1999

Akbar SMF, Abe M, Masumoto T, Horiike N, Onji M (1999) Mechanism of action of vaccine therapy in murine hepatitis B virus carriers: vaccine-induced activation of antigen presenting dendritic cells. J Hepatol 30:755–764

Akbar SMF, Horiike N, Onji M (1999) Prognostic importance of antigen-presenting dendritic cells during vaccine therapy in a murine hepatitis B virus carrier. Immunology 96:68–108 **(Fig. 3.3, Fig. 3.4)**

Akbar SMF, Kajino K, Tanimoto K, Yamamura K, Onji M, Hino O (1999) Unique features of dendritic cells in IFN-γ transgenic mice: relevance to cancer development and therapeutic implications. Biochem Biophys Res Commun 259:294–299

Akbar SMF, Onji M, Hino O (1999) Antigen-presenting dendritic cells in the pathogenesis and therapy of cancer. In: SG Pandalai (Ed.) Recent Research Development in Cancer. Research Signpost, Trivandram, India, pp 229–236

Akbar SMF, Yamamoto K, Abe M, Ninomiya T, Tanimoto K, Masumoto T, Michitaka K, Horiike N, Onji M (1999) Potent synergistic effect of sho-saiko-to, a herbal medicine, during vaccine therapy in a murine model of hepatitis B virus carrier. Eur J Clin Invest 29:786–792

Ninomiya T, Akbar SMF, Masumoto T, Horiike N, Onji M (1999) Dendritic cells with immature phenotype and defective function in the peripheral blood from patients with hepatocellular carcinoma. J Hepatol 31:323–331

Onji M, Akbar SMF, Hiasa Y, Masumoto T, Horiike N, Michitaka K (1999) Intrahepatic dendritic cells. Prog Hepatol 5:15–22

Shinomiya M, Akbar SMF, Sinomiya H, Onji M (1999) Transfer of dendritic cells (DC) ex vivo stimulated with interferon-gamma (IFN-γ) down-modulates autoimmune diabetes in non-obese diabetic (NOD) mice. Clin Exp Immunol 117:38–43

Tamaru M, Matsuura B, Onji M (1999) Dendritic cells produce interleukin-12 in hyperthyroid mice. Eur J Endocrinol 141:625–629

Tanimoto K, Akbar SMF, Michitaka K, Onji M (1999) Immunohistochemical localization of antigen presenting cells in liver from patients with primary biliary cirrhosis: highly restricted distribution of CD83-positive activated dendritic cells. Pathol Res Pract 195:157–162 **(Fig. 5.3)**

2000

Akbar SMF, Onji M (2000) Immune therapies for chronic hepatitis B virus carrier: role of recently developed vaccine therapy and traditional Chinese herbal medicine (sho-saiko-to). Cent Eur J Immunol 25:37–42

Chen S, Akbar SMF, Tanimoto K, Ninomiya T, Iuchi H, Michitaka K, Horiike N, Onji M (2000) Absence of CD83-positive mature and activated dendritic cells at cancer nodules from patients with hepatocellular carcinoma: relevance to hepatocarcinogenesis. Cancer Lett 148:49–57 **(Fig. 6.5)**

Masumoto T, Yamamoto K, Abe M, Akbar SMF, Onji M (2000) Role of dendritic cells in patients with primary biliary cirrhosis. Autoimmune Liver Disease: Its Recent Advances, Tokyo, Elsevier Science B.V. 149–155

Ninomiya T, Matsui H, Akbar SMF, Murakami H, Onji M (2000) Localization and characterization of antigen-presenting dendritic cells in the gastric mucosa of murine and human autoimmune gastritis. Eur J Clin Invest 30:350–358 **(Fig 5.1)**

Okazaki A, Tanimoto K, Akbar SMF, Ninomiya T, Kumagi T, Abe M, Hiasa Y, Masumoto T, Michitaka K, Horiike N, Onji M (2000) Expression of inducible nitric oxide synthase on antigen-presenting cells in patients with primary biliary cirrhosis. Dendritic Cells 10: 23–24 **(Fig. 5.5)**

Shinomiya M, Nadano S, Shinomiya H, Onji M (2000) In situ characterization of dendritic cells occurring in the islets of nonobese diabetic mice during the development of insulitis. Pancreas 20:290–296

2001

Abe M, Akbar SMF, Horiike N, Onji M (2001) Induction of cytokine production and proliferation of memory lymphocytes by murine liver dendritic cell progenitors: role of these progenitors as immunogenic resident antigen-presenting cells in the liver. J Hepatol 34:67–71

Akbar SMF, Horiike N, Onji M, Hino O (2001) Dendritic cells and chronic hepatitis virus-carriers. Intervirology 44:199–208

Akbar SMF, Yamamoto K, Miyakawa H, Ninomiya T, Abe M, Hiasa Y, Masumoto T, Horiike N, Onji M (2001) Peripheral blood T-cell responses to pyruvate dehydrogenase complex in primary biliary cirrhosis: role of antigen-presenting dendritic cells: Eur J Clin Invest 31:639–646

Ikeda Y, Akbar SMF, Matsui H, Onji M (2001) Characterization of antigen-presenting dendritic cells in the peripheral blood and colonic mucosa of patients with ulcerative colitis. Eur J Gastroenterol Hepatol 13:841–850 **(Fig. 5.3)**

Murakami H, Akbar SMF, Matsui H, Onji M (2001) Macrophage migration inhibitory factor in the sera and at the colonic mucosa in patients with ulcerative colitis: clinical implications and pathogenic significance. Eur J Clin Invest 31:337–343

Oka Y, Akbar SMF, Horiike N, Joko K, Onji M (2001) Mechanism and therapeutic potential of DNA-based immunization against the envelope proteins of hepatitis B virus in normal and transgenic mice. Immunology 103:90–97 **(Fig. 3.4)**

Onji M, Akbar SMF, Horiike N (2001) Dendritic cell-based immunotherapy for hepatocellular carcinoma. J Gastroenterol 36:794–797

Tanimoto K, Akbar SMF, Michitaka K, Horiike N, Onji M (2001) Antigen-presenting cells at the liver tissue in patients with chronic viral liver diseases: CD83-positive mature dendritic cells at the vicinity of focal and confluent necrosis. Hepatol Res 21:117–125

2002

Abe M, Kajino K, Akbar SMF, Yamamura K, Onji M, Hino O (2002) Loss of immunogenicity of liver dendritic cells from mouse with chronic hepatitis. Int J Mol Med 9:71–76

Hiasa Y, Akbar SMF, Abe M, Michitaka K, Horiike N, Onji M (2002) Dendritic cell subtypes in autoimmune liver diseases: decreased expression of HLA DR and CD123 on type 2 dendritic cells. Hepatol Res 22:241–249

Horiike N, Akbar SMF, Ninomiya T, Abe M, Michitaka K, Onji M (2002) Activation and maturation of antigen-presenting dendritic cells during vaccine therapy in patients with chronic hepatitis due to hepatitis B virus. Hepatol Res 23:38–47 **(Fig. 3.5)**

Ikeda Y, Akbar SMF, Matsui H, Onji M (2002) Antigen-presenting dendritic cells in ulcerative colitis. J Gastroenterol 37:53–55

Murakami H, Akbar SMF, Matsui H, Horiike N, Onji M (2002) Macrophage migration inhibitory factor activates antigen-presenting dendritic cells and induces inflammatory cytokines in ulcerative colitis. Clin Exp Immunol 128:504–510

2003

Abe M, Akbar SMF, Horiike N, Onji M (2003) Inability of liver dendritic cells from mouse with experimental hepatitis to process and present specific antigens. Hepatol Res 26: 61–67

Abe M, Akbar SMF, Horiike N, Onji M (2003) Glycyrrhizin enhances interleukin-10 production from liver dendritic cells in mice with hepatitis. J Gastroenterol (in press)

Abe M, Akbar SMF, Matsuura B, Horiike N, Onji M (2003) Defective antigen-presenting capacity of murine dendritic cells during starvation. Nutrition 19:265–269

Akbar SMF, Furukawa S, Abe M, Michitaka K, Chen Y, Horiike N, Onji M. Production, therapeutic effect and mechanism of action of a vaccine containing antigen-pulsed dendritic cells for treatment of chronic hepatitis B virus infection. Hepatology 2002; 36 (suppl): 301A.

Arima S, Akbar SMF, Michitaka K, Horiike N, Nuriya H, Kohara M, Onji M (2003) Impaired function of antigen-presenting dendritic cells in patients with chronic hepatitis B: localization of HBV DNA and HBV RNA in blood DC by in situ hybridization. Int J Mol Med 11:169–174 **(Fig. 3.2)**

Ikeda Y, Akbar SMF, Matsui H, Murakami H, Onji M (2003) Depletion and decreased function of antigen-presenting dendritic cells caused by lymphocytapheresis in ulcerative colitis. Dis Colon Rectum 46:521–528 **(Fig. 5.6)**

Kumagi T, Akbar SMG, Horiike N, Onji M (in press). Increased survival and decreased tumor size due to intratumoral injection of ethanol followed by administration of immature dendritic cells. Int J Oncol. **(Fig. 6.8)**

Tsubouchi E, Horiike N, Akbar SMF, Matsuura B, Michitaka K, Abe M, Hiasa Y, Onji M (suppl). Infection and dysfunction of circulating dendritic cells in chronic hepatitis C virus infection: activation of dendritic cells by antiviral therapy. Hepatology 2002; 36; 226A

Subject Index

Author

Morikazu Onji, M.D., Ph.D.
Curriculum Vitae

Date of Birth:	February 13, 1948
Place of Birth:	Ehime, Japan
March 1973	Graduated from Kagoshima University School of Medicine
May 1973	Resident, The First Department of Internal Medicine, Okayama University, Medical School
June 1974	Medical Staff in Internal Medicine, Saiseikai Imabari Hospital
April 1976	Clinical and Research Fellow, The First Department of Biochemistry, Osaka City Medical School
April 1977	Assistant Professor, The Third Department of Internal Medicine, Ehime University School of Medicine
November 1984	Ph.D. (Doctor of Medical Science) Ehime University
May 1985	Associate Professor (Lecturer), The Third Department of Internal Medicine, Ehime University
January 1986	Research Fellow, Royal Free Hospital, London University
May 1994–present	Professor and Chairman, The Third Department of Internal Medicine, Ehime University
April 2000–present	Head, Endoscopy Center, Ehime University Hospital
April 2000–present	Deputy Director, Ehime University Hospital

Award

1988 Young Investigation Award from the Japan Society of Hepatology
1988 Award from the Kanae Foundation for Life and Socio-Medical Science
1991 Investigator's Award from the Japan Gastroenterological Endoscopy Society
1992 Investigator's Award from the Foundation for Viral Hepatitis Research

Society Membership

American Association for the Study of Liver Diseases (AASLD)
European Association for the Study of the Liver (EASL)
International Association for the Study of the Liver (IASL)
Asian Pacific Association for the Study of the Liver (APASL)
Japanese Society of Gastroenterology (Member of Council)
Japan Society of Hepatology (Member of Council)
Liver Cancer Study Group of Japan (Member of Council)
Japan Gastroenterological Endoscopy Society (Member of Council)
Japanese Society of Allergology (Member of Council)
Japanese Society of Mucosal Immunology (Executive Board Member)
Japan Diabetic Society (Member of Council)
Japan Society of Metabolism and Clinical Nutrition (Executive Board Member)

Research Specialties
1) Liver immunology; autoimmune liver diseases, the viral hepatitis B and C
2) Dendritic cells in digestive organs
3) Macroscopic (laparoscopic) and microscopic study of the liver

Contributors

Sk. Md. Fazle Akbar, MBBS, Ph.D.
1980   Medical Graduate, Rajshahi Medical College, Bangladesh
1985   Evaluator, Communicable Disease Control, D/G Health, Bangladesh
1993   Ph.D. in Medical Science, Ehime University, Ehime, Japan
1993   Research Assistant, Institute of Postgraduate Medicine & Research, Dhaka, Bangladesh
1994   Postdoctoral Fellow, Ehime University School of Medicine, Japan
1996   Assistant Professor, Department of Hygiene, Ehime University School of Medicine, Japan
1998   Assistant Professor, Third Department of Internal Medicine, Ehime University School of Medicine, Japan

Norio Horiike, M.D., Ph.D.
1978   Medical Graduate, Kagoshima University School of Medicine, Japan
1978   Resident, Third Department of Internal Medicine, Ehime University School of Medicine, Japan
1984   Assistant Professor, Third Department of Internal Medicine, Ehime University School of Medicine, Japan
1989   Postdoctoral Fellow, Fox Chase Cancer Center, Philadelphia, U.S.A.
1995   Associate Professor, Third Department of Internal Medicine, Ehime University School of Medicine, Japan